101 Healthiest Foods

101 Healthiest Foods

A Quick and Easy Guide
to the Fruits, Vegetables,
Carbs and Proteins
That Can Save Your Life

Dr. Joanna McMillan Price and Judy Davie

Ulysses Press

Published in the U.S. by
Ulysses Press
P.O. Box 3440
Berkeley, CA 94703
www.ulyssespress.com

First published as *Star Foods* in Australia in 2008 by ABC Books.

ISBN: 978-1-56975-666-9
Library of Congress Control Number 2008911702

Acquisitions Editor: Nick Denton-Brown
Managing Editor: Claire Chun
U.S. Editor: Lauren Harrison
Proofreader: Abigail Reser
Design and layout: what!design @ whatweb.com
Cover photo: istockphoto.com

Printed in Canada by Webcom

10 9 8 7 6 5 4 3 2 1

Distributed by Publishers Group West

NOTE TO READERS

This book has been written and published strictly for informational and educational purposes only. It is not intended to serve as medical advice or to be any form of medical treatment. You should always consult your physician before altering or changing any aspect of your medical treatment and/or undertaking a diet regimen, including the guidelines as described in this book. Do not stop or change any prescription medications without the guidance and advice of your physician. Any use of the information in this book is made on the reader's good judgment after consulting with his or her physician and is the reader's sole responsibility. This book is not intended to diagnose or treat any medical condition and is not a substitute for a physician.

CONTENTS

INTRODUCTION

What you eat has the power to influence the way you look, how you feel, how much energy you have, your ability to perform mental tasks, your ability to exercise, and your general state of happiness — and that's before we even start to talk about lowering your risk of chronic disease.

Changing to a healthier diet is about being proactive and responsible for your own health and vitality. It's about preventing disease rather than contributing to it. If you speak to anyone who's given up smoking only to start again weeks, months, or years later, the chances are they'll tell you that somewhere in the back of their mind they believed they would smoke again. Likewise, anyone who goes "on a diet" expects to resume their normal eating habits as soon as the diet is over. That is not what this book is about.

The word "diet" has been misused for too long. It is associated with weight loss and conjures up feelings of guilt, deprivation, and misery. But what "diet" really means, quite simply, is the food you eat on a day-to-day basis. It is our diet that has an impact on our health and well-being, and not individual foods or whole food groups. And while disease is influenced by many factors out of our control (genetics being the most obvious example), diet plays an enormous role and is an area we can control.

To be healthy, change your eating habits forever

To be healthy, you have to change your eating habits forever. These are words many of us don't want to hear but they speak the truth. Whether you like it or not, if you want to be healthy and free from the rollercoaster of diet-related mental purgatory, you have no choice but to retrain your eating habits, improve your culinary skills, and educate your children to do the same.

The difficulty is in knowing what changes you should make. Who do you believe when barely a day goes by without mention of health scares, obesity problems, and miracle cures or concerns about single foods — all information that is usually superseded by something else? It's ludicrous to expect a single food to cure cancer, prevent heart disease, or manage diabetes, and similarly unfair to label any single food as the cause of disease or weight gain. Tomatoes alone won't prevent cancer, nor will a few sweet foods give you diabetes. A sirloin steak won't give you colon cancer, and a potato now and again won't make you fat, even if it is fried. But neither is it fair to categorize entire food groups as good or bad. History has, time and again, shown us that extreme diets that eliminate entire food groups inevitably lead to unhealthy attitudes toward food, weight problems, and poor health. Just as important, such diets are particularly unpalatable, hard to sustain, unsociable, and just not fun.

While the science of nutrition gets incredibly complicated as it battles out the intricacies of how foods and drinks affect our health, the conclusions in broader terms are really quite simple and clear.

A fresh, natural diet including a large variety of minimally processed foods, encompassing every food group, is the safest and healthiest way to eat.

The organic debate

Some people believe that unless it's 100 percent organic, from the producer direct to the customer, it's not healthy. Others want the convenience of packaged foods and rely on scientific-sounding supplements to fill any gaps. We take the middle ground. If you want to go organic, that's great. Organic farming helps to protect our planet in a number of ways, not least by reducing the number of chemicals in the air and earth. While there is ongoing scientific debate over the nutritional differences between organic and conventional produce, a European study headed by Newcastle University in the UK has just released findings that show significantly higher levels of particular nutrients, including antioxidants, in organic produce. For example they found that the levels of antioxidants in organic milk were up to 90 percent higher than conventional milk and up to 40 percent more antioxidants were found in organic vegetables than conventional ones. With this building nutritional evidence and the growing concern over our environment there is no question that buying organic is the ideal. However, the fact is that the substantial price hike from conventional to organic means choosing the latter is simply not achievable for many. We hope in time this situation changes, but in the meantime what we do know is that fresh produce, eaten (or frozen) within as short a time frame as possible, does contain more nutrients than packaged or processed produce whether it is organic or not. You may also want to consider the environmental implications of fossil fuels burned to transport organic "health foods" from the other side of the world. We therefore recommend eating locally grown food in season as much as possible — if you can afford to support our organic farmers, even better.

Unfortunately, the organic label has also become a bit of a marketing ploy. For example, a processed breakfast cereal remains a processed breakfast cereal — the fact that it is made from organic ingredients doesn't really make it any better for us. Be careful not to assume a product is healthy just because it is organic. (That said, organic products don't contain artificial preservatives, additives, or colors, and this is certainly advantageous.)

The bottom line is there is much that you can do to improve your diet and your health that will have a far bigger impact than making the leap to organics. There is little point in spending the extra money on organics if you continue to smoke socially on the weekend, continue to eat too few plant foods and too many packaged foods, or continue to spend too many hours sitting on your bottom.

Put organics into perspective. Think of a ladder of dietary changes you could make to improve your health with organics right at the top. You can choose to take that final step and eat nothing but organic and manage your life around that ideal, or come down a few notches and simply make the best choices that you can. Certainly climb as high as you can, but not to the point where you're likely to fall. Only make changes that you can reasonably keep up forever. This makes it easier, do-able, and sustainable.

About this book

This book pulls together scientific facts, assumptions, and practical applications. It brings you the latest information from research in the field of nutritional science while recognizing that there's still a lot we don't know. To this end, our ranking of foods is based on fact as far as is possible, but by necessity we have often had to make an educated decision based on the balance of evidence to date. Our ideas are not intended to be set in stone, but to provide you with the skills to create a healthy diet that works with your lifestyle and eating preferences.

Our goal is to guide you toward the foods with the potential to give you more bang for your buck while steering you away from those that may do more harm than good. To this end, we have ranked foods based on their merits and/or demerits and created divisions within each food category. Think of the foods you choose to eat as players on your healthy eating team. Choosing the best players is your best chance of achieving a winning team and therefore a winning diet. The prize is immediate in the way you will look and feel and in maximizing your chances of achieving and maintaining good health in both the short and long term.

We know that if you eat a wide range of foods from each food group you'll feel good, but you'll feel fabulous if you select the top-ranking items from each food group as often as possible. We truly believe there are many people who don't know how good they could look and feel if only they ate better. Experience this for yourself and we guarantee that over time you will increasingly want to eat more of the foods from the top categories, and fewer of the foods from the bottom, not because we tell you they are better, but because you feel and look better when you choose to eat this way.

This is not a book about deprivation or banning foods. It's not a book to make you feel guilty when you eat or make you a slave to the kitchen forever. Enjoying food is a prerequisite to healthy eating. You need to take pleasure in all aspects of food — from selecting good quality produce, preparing it (quickly most of the time) in delicious ways, and savoring your efforts. Without a passion for the process, your dietary changes will be unsustainable and you'll soon revert to old habits. Suspend disbelief, open your mind to believe you can eat healthily, enjoy your food, and relish in the numerous health benefits as a result.

In short, our aim is to teach you:

- What to eat — selecting the best of the best, the 5-star foods

- Why some foods are better than others — the science behind the food

- How to put it all together with easy, quick, healthy, and delicious recipes and tips.

Work with the information in this book to find a diet that makes you feel much better than you do now: a diet that gives you more energy than you currently have and allows you to live a fuller life than you are living, a diet that you enjoy, that's easy to stick to, and one you feel you can stay on forever.

Part 1:
101 Healthiest Foods

THE BIG PICTURE — RETHINKING THE FOOD PYRAMID

Before we talk about each food group, it is helpful to think about the role food groups play in our overall diet. This is the big picture and it is good to have it in your head before getting down to the best individual food choices.

You'll notice that our food pyramid in Figure 1.1 on page 4 differs from the traditional food pyramid. Old-school thinking placed the carbohydrate-rich grain foods — such as bread, rice, and pasta — along with vegetables and fruits at the base. This was intended to encourage us toward a low-fat, high-carbohydrate diet. Yet, as the obesity epidemic threatens to engulf us, this pyramid is failing us fast. While modern diets tend to be energy dense and nutrient poor, leading to weight gain and ill health, our revamped food pyramid is designed to reverse this. It will guide you toward a diet that gives you more bang for your buck, a diet that is nutrient dense but energy saving. It is a back-to-nature approach, reflecting the way we were designed to eat, and factors in the latest nutrition research.

Vegetables and fruits form the base. For very few calories, vegetables and fruits provide an incredible wealth of essential nutrients. In essence, this means you can afford to eat a lot more of these foods than any other.

On the second level you'll find a flexible line between the more energy-dense, protein-rich, and carb-rich foods. So long as you eat the minimum from each group, you can move this line to have more protein and fewer carbohydrates, or vice versa. How much of each you choose to eat will depend largely on factors such as your food preferences, exercise levels, and body type.

Near the top of the pyramid lie the fat-rich foods. Because these foods are energy dense, the volume of them we eat needs to be less; but because they contain many essential nutrients not found in other foods (not to mention the taste and flavor they impart) they must be included in your daily diet.

And, finally, at the tip of the pyramid are the treats. Treats are the foods and drinks that really give you pleasure but don't add much in the way of nutrients and tend to be loaded with calories. Because treats are energy dense and nutrient poor they are the polar opposite of vegetables and fruits at the base of the pyramid.

Examples of treats include chocolates, lollipops, burgers, gin and tonics, or whatever else you feel you couldn't live without, regardless of what we say. And neither should you have to. As long as you remember the positioning of treats in the food pyramid and eat them in that proportion so that the bulk of your diet is packed full of 5-star foods, it really doesn't matter much what makes up this small space. That said, we will of course try to guide you toward the healthiest treats possible!

Why do we need to eat from each of these food groups? Well it's quite simply this — each food group provides a different set of nutrients and has a special purpose. Without some of each, your body cannot perform at its best and, sooner or later, you'll feel the effect. Perhaps you don't eat enough vegetables and fruits, and suffer from more colds and flus than you need to; or you've cut out carbs to try to lose weight and find yourself constipated and unable to concentrate. You may have chosen to cut out meat, can't cook fish, and don't understand tofu, but you always feel tired, your spirits are low, and you never feel fully satisfied after meals. Or you may be battling with your weight on a low-fat diet and have dry skin, a foul temper, and an unbearable craving for a giant block of chocolate. The solution is to eat more different kinds of foods, not fewer. Broaden your palate to include foods from each of our food groups in the proportions illustrated in the pyramid.

There is no one food that will help you achieve great health — it is the collective power of everything you eat that produces results. Figure 1.2 on page 5 illustrates the ideal food pyramid and the role of each food group within it.

Remember, it's important to eat for pleasure, but also to eat well. You need to understand which foods are best for your body and how to choose the ones that will bring you the most physical and emotional satisfaction. Fresh vegetables and fruits are your defense against infections and chronic disease. They'll protect you from ill health and help you get on with life. Proteins strengthen and maintain the body, while carbohydrates give you the energy and determination to go strong all day and recharge as you sleep at night. Fats play a strategic role in your diet — they should never be left out, but you need to know how to use them correctly. And remember, treats are a great way to celebrate successes, but make sure that those little indulgences don't send you all the way back square one on your journey toward better health.

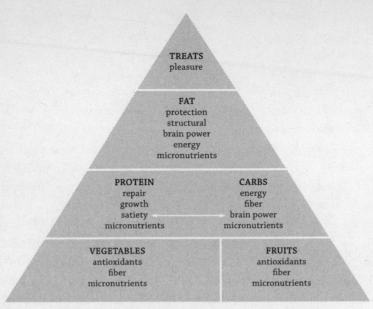

FIGURE 1.1: A new way of thinking about the food pyramid

To help you make the best choices that will keep your body and mind strong, we rank foods within each of the food groups into five divisions:

5-STAR FOODS ☆ ☆ ☆ ☆ ☆ — These are the very best foods you can choose. They give our bodies something extra, so include as many of these in your diet as possible.

4-STAR FOODS ☆ ☆ ☆ ☆ — These are good, solid choices and can happily be included in your daily diet.

3-STAR FOODS ☆ ☆ ☆ — These are hearty, reliable foods that may lack stand-out quality but nevertheless have some merit and few flaws.

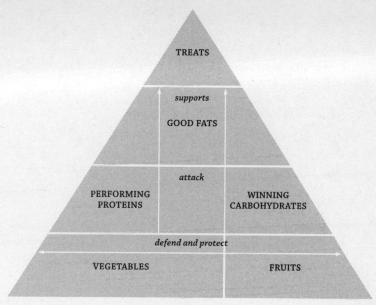

FIGURE 1.2: The winning team

2-STAR FOODS ☆ ☆ — You shouldn't eat these foods every day, but they're all right. These are choices with some black marks to their name, but they have some value — consider them "now and then" foods.

1-STAR FOODS ☆ — If you can avoid them, you should try to never eat these foods. They have little, if anything, nutritional to offer while potentially doing much harm if consumed too often. Choose them rarely, if at all. However, if they happen to be a food you really, really love, indulging *every now and then* will do no harm in the overall scheme of things.

How well are you eating now?

To give yourself an idea about how well you are currently eating, answer our quick quiz. You can then prioritize the changes you need to make to improve your diet. Check the statements that are true today.

VEGETABLES AND FRUITS

- I eat fewer than five servings of different vegetables a day.
- I don't eat fresh green leafy vegetables every day.
- I often eat potatoes or potato products.
- I eat fewer vegetables than any other food group each day.
- I eat fewer than two pieces of different fruit each day.
- I tend to eat the same vegetables and fruits every week.
- I eat fewer vegetables than fruits.

If you checked any of the above, your diet is likely to be lacking nutritional value. To improve your performance, turn to page 9 and read about vegetables and fruits.

GRAINS, CEREALS, AND LEGUMES (CARBOHYDRATE-RICH FOODS)

- I rarely choose foods high in fiber.
- I am often hungry an hour or two after meals and find it hard not to snack between meals.
- I regularly eat processed or refined carbohydrates (white breads, crackers, breakfast cereals).
- I rarely eat legumes (beans, chickpeas, kidney beans, lentils).
- I rarely choose whole-grain products.
- I often avoid carbohydrates to try to lose weight.

If you checked any of the above, your diet is likely to be lacking nutritional value. To improve your performance, turn to page 29 and read about carbohydrates.

MEAT, SEAFOOD, DAIRY, EGGS, AND LEGUMES (PROTEIN-RICH FOODS)

- I eat fish or seafood less than twice a week.

- I rarely choose lean cuts of meat and poultry.

- I don't know how to combine plant foods to meet my protein needs.

- I rarely choose low-fat dairy products (or soy alternatives).

- I don't always include a protein source in every meal (from animals or plants).

- I regularly eat processed meat (salami, sliced cold meats, sausages).

If you checked any of the above, your diet is likely to be lacking nutritional value. To improve your performance, turn to page 51 and read about proteins.

OILS, NUTS, AND SEEDS (FAT-RICH FOODS)

- I eat deep-fried foods more than once a week.

- I rarely eat nuts and/or seeds.

- I use butter and/or margarine.

- I don't know which oils to use for different cooking applications.

- I eat oily fish less than twice a week.

- I love fast food and eat it regularly.

- I usually eat the skin and fat on meat and poultry.

If you checked any of the above, your diet is likely to be lacking nutritional value. To improve your performance turn, to page 72 and read about fats.

DRINKS

- I drink more than 2 standard drinks a day (standard drink = 6 oz. wine, 8 oz. beer, 1 oz. liquor).

- I rarely choose to drink plain water.

- I regularly drink fruit juice and keep cartons in the fridge at home.

- I drink alcohol almost every night.

- I often drink coffee or tea but I'm not sure if I should limit my intake of these.

- I often drink sweetened fizzy drinks or diet drinks on their own or as an alcoholic mixer.

If you checked any of the above, your diet is likely to be lacking nutritional value. To improve your performance, turn to page 92 and read about drinks.

TREATS

- I eat a lot of packaged food (cakes, cookies, chips, crackers, and other snack foods).

- I eat sweet treats more than three times a week.

- I often buy candy.

- I often have treats in place of a proper meal.

If you checked any of the above, your diet is likely to be lacking nutritional value. To improve your performance, turn to page 96 and read about treats.

VEGETABLES AND FRUITS

WORLD'S HEALTHIEST VEGETABLES
☆ ☆ ☆ ☆ ☆

Asparagus

The Cabbage Family (including Asian greens, broccoli and broccolini, Brussels sprouts, dark green cabbage, red cabbage)

Dark Green Leafy Vegetables (including curly kale, endive, arugula, spinach, and watercress)

Bell Peppers and Chili Peppers

Globe Artichokes

Mushrooms

The Onion Family (including garlic, onions, leeks, green onions, and shallots)

Parsley

Peas — Green and Sugar Snap/Snow Peas

Tomatoes

WORLD'S HEALTHIEST FRUITS

☆ ☆ ☆ ☆ ☆

Apricots, Fresh and Dried

Avocados

Berries (including blueberries, blackberries, cranberries, raspberries, and strawberries)

Cantaloupe

Citrus Fruit (including grapefruit, pink grapefruit, kumquats, oranges)

Guavas

Kiwifruit

Mangoes

Papayas

Passion Fruit

Persimmons

Pomegranates

Prunes

How many times have you heard the saying "eat more fruits and veggies"? By now it no doubt seems a boring and tired old adage started by your mother and is just a continuing nag to perpetuate with your own kids. But where there is smoke there is fire and, while the world of nutritional science remains controversial about many things, this message has stood the test of time.

The current recommendation in America is to eat five a day; but the truth is this is almost certainly not the optimum, it's just that this is what is considered achievable given that the vast majority of us fail to even come close to this. You would be hard pressed to find a nutrition expert anywhere in the world who would not agree that one of the most positive things we can do for our health is to up our intake of vegetables and fruits. So think of the five a day as the minimum and get serious about eating more of these fabulous foods.

Fruit has taken a bashing following the popularity of low-carb diets, and many people believe fruit is bad for them because it contains sugar. Perhaps it is the belief that something that tastes so good cannot possibly be good for us. Thankfully, that is not true as we hope to prove to you in this book. A healthy diet is good for the body, the mind and the taste buds. Sugar in fruit is not the same as foods containing a lot of added refined sugar. The term "sugar" just means short-chain or single carbohydrates — for example, glucose is the type of sugar that circulates in our bloodstream, fructose is found in fruit, lactose is found in milk, and sucrose is the type of sugar we find in packet or table sugar. Sugar is not necessarily bad and, in many cases, is a very good source of energy. The key point is not whether there is sugar present in a food, but whether that sugar is intrinsic to the food (as in the case of fruit and milk) or added to the food (as in many processed foods).

Most fruits have a low glycemic index (GI) and this means that the sugars present are slowly absorbed, having a smaller and steadier effect on your blood-sugar levels than many other foods that contain little or no sugar, such as white bread or rice. Fruits are also packed with fiber, antioxidants, and other nutrients our bodies need. What's more, humans have eaten fruits (and vegetables) throughout history. It doesn't make sense that low-carb diets exclude these wonderful, naturally sweet foods, while simultaneously promoting the use of processed protein powders and manufactured supplements! We must stop demonizing foods based on their carb (or fat) content and look at the bigger picture.

You'll notice we always refer to "vegetables and fruits" rather than the usual "fruits and vegetables." The reason is that we find it far easier to get people eating more fruit because most fruit is sweet and we have an inherent liking for sweet tastes. It tends to be vegetables that are left behind and these are 5-star foods in our dietary defense against disease and being overweight. While it's possible to eat more fruit than you really need, it is almost impossible to do the same with vegetables. This is the one food group where you have carte blanche to load your plate and dig in.

Five reasons for eating more vegetables and fruits

1. Vegetables and fruits are packed with a whole host of antioxidants that fight disease and slow the aging process.

2. Vegetables and fruits provide us with numerous essential vitamins and minerals we need to function and perform at our peak.

3. Most vegetables and fruits have a low energy density so, by replacing more energy-dense foods in your diet, they can help with weight control.

4. Vegetables and fruits provide considerable amounts of fiber and this helps to keep your digestive system healthy, slow blood sugar responses, and keep your cholesterol levels in check.

5. Good, quality vegetables and fruits taste delicious! They add texture, color, flavor, and aroma to dishes when used in the right way.

Ways to eat more

There are many ways to incorporate more vegetables and fruits into your diet. Here are some suggestions to get you started:

- If you can't make it regularly to the grocery store, use an online company that delivers direct to your door. Many websites now deliver direct from the market, rather than via the major supermarkets, ensuring better quality and freshness.

- Keep the freezer stocked with a selection of vegetables including corn cobs, green peas, spinach, and stir-fry variety packs. Frozen fruit can also be a great option; for example, frozen berries work well and are often a lot less expensive than fresh. Freezing preserves the nutrient content and also negates the need for added preservatives.

- Add vegetables into dishes such as stews, casseroles, curries, and pasta sauces.

- Stuff sandwiches and wraps with extra salad fillings.

- Have a side salad with your meal whenever possible.
- Keep a fruit bowl on your desk and/or at home and grab a piece when you feel hungry between meals or crave something sweet.

World's Healthiest Vegetables ☆ ☆ ☆ ☆ ☆

ASPARAGUS

In Scotland when we were growing up, asparagus was a rare treat because this wonderful vegetable was hard to come by and it was very expensive. In fact, it was one of the only vegetables to be thought of as a treat and one we all savored and asked for more of. Today, asparagus is far more widely available, although still relatively expensive because of the practicalities involved in growing it in large quantities. However, it is worth every penny. Asparagus is an excellent source of fiber, vitamin A, vitamin C, vitamin K, thiamin, riboflavin, niacin, folate, iron, phosphorus, potassium, copper, and manganese. Depending on where it is grown, it can also be an excellent source of the antioxidant mineral selenium. Asparagus also contains:

- **SAPONINS** — compounds thought to prevent heart disease by helping to reduce blood cholesterol levels.

- **VITAMIN B6** — known for its role in converting food into energy in the body, but this vitamin may also help to reduce PMS and the nausea of early pregnancy. (Be wary of consuming vitamin B6 supplements to treat PMS — too much is toxic and can affect nerve function. Eat your asparagus instead and you can never overdo it!)

- **RUTIN** — an antioxidant from the bioflavonoid family that plays an important role in strengthening blood vessels. Rutin may therefore be helpful if you have varicose veins, high blood pressure, poor circulation, or broken capillaries.

THE CABBAGE FAMILY

Technically called the *Brassica* (genus) or Cruciferous (family) vegetables, the cabbage family includes broccoli, broccolini, cauliflower, Brussels sprouts, bok choy, and all varieties of cabbage (dark green cabbages, such as savoy, and red cabbage are particularly nutrient rich). Unfortunately, many of us have been scarred by memories of being forced to eat pale, lifeless, overcooked cabbage or bitter Brussels sprouts and have vowed never to go there again. We hope to convince you otherwise and tempt you back to these fabulous foods.

The cabbage family has been the source of numerous studies after research showed that those who ate the most of these vegetables had lower incidence of some cancers, particularly colon cancer. In fact, one of the first studies Joanna worked on looked at how broccoli affected the susceptibility of cells lining the colon to carcinogenic damage. The findings were that eating raw broccoli provided the most protection for the colon, whereas eating the cooked vegetable got more antioxidants into the bloodstream where they could potentially prevent damage elsewhere in the body (Ratcliffe et al, 2000). In other words, there were different benefits associated with eating the raw and cooked vegetable. You may have assumed eating raw food is always better (many diet books have told us so) but, in fact, the science tells us otherwise. By eating your veggies in both raw and cooked forms, you maximize your body's defenses. Raw broccoli florets are deliciously crunchy tossed in a mixed salad, while raw cabbage is a culinary classic in coleslaw and can be fabulously nutritious when prepared in the right way (try Judy's version on page 179 as part of the recipe "Lentil & Freekeh Patties with Coleslaw"). Broccoli, broccolini, and cauliflower all make great additions to a stir-fry, curry, or casserole.

The vegetables chart table (page 100) gives you an overview of the nutrients found in each type of Cruciferous vegetable but, as a family, the key factors are:

A whole host of phytochemicals including flavonoids, dithiolthiones, glucosinolates, isothiocyanates, sulforaphane, and indoles. Forget about the confusing names, suffice to say that these compounds fight cancer and/or heart disease and probably a whole lot more. We also give you the names as a good illustration of how supplement antioxidant pills cannot provide nearly the number of goodies found in real food.

- **LUTEIN** — one of the carotenoid family of antioxidants, thought to have various benefits for our health. The strongest evidence is for its role in eye health where, along with its partner zeaxanthin, it has been linked to a reduced risk of age-related macular degeneration (AMD), a major cause of vision loss. Lutein may also play a role in maintaining healthy skin, in part by providing some protection against damage from sunlight. At least one study has shown lutein can slow down atherosclerosis (the plaque build-up in the arteries that can eventually cause a heart attack). Finally, lutein is part of the team of antioxidants thought to be important in reducing the risk of certain cancers.

- **ANTHOCYANINS** — red/purple pigments found in red cabbage. They are powerful antioxidants that contribute to the body's defense against free-radical damage.

- **INSOLUBLE FIBER** — needed to keep the stomach contents moving and prevent constipation.

- **FOLATE** — a B vitamin; a good intake can reduce your heart disease risk. If you are planning to have a baby, folate reduces the risk of neural tube defects.

- **VITAMIN C** — one of the key antioxidants, also important for maintaining a healthy, strong immune system. Since vitamin C is easily destroyed in cooking and is lost during storage, aim to include a few raw sources or cook only lightly and eat soon after purchase.

- **POTASSIUM** — important for keeping blood pressure in check.

- **VITAMIN K** — for healthy blood clotting. Broccoli and Brussels sprouts are particularly rich in this vitamin.

BELL PEPPERS AND CHILI PEPPERS

Bell peppers of all colors and chilies are 5-star foods because they are packed with nutrients that help to protect us from heart disease and cancers and are great for eye health. In particular they contain:

- **BETA-CAROTENE** — an antioxidant especially rich in red bell pepper. Beta-carotene can also be converted to vitamin A which, among other things, is essential for good vision. Two other carotenoids also important for eye health are lutein and zeaxanthin, found in abundance in red and orange bell peppers.

- **VITAMIN C** — a major antioxidant and, among its many functions, is essential for good immune function and healthy, glowing skin. Since this vitamin is easily destroyed by cooking, try to eat it raw some of the time — for example chop raw bell pepper into your salad.

- **CAPSAICIN** — the compound responsible for the heat in chilies. If you like it hot (and the hotter the chili, the greater the capsaicin content) the good news is that capsaicin has a number of potential benefits: It can ease nasal congestion, encourage cancer cell death, detoxify cancer-causing compounds, and boost your metabolism.

- **FIBER** — necessary for good digestive function and soluble fiber can help to reduce blood cholesterol levels. The fiber is found mostly in the skin, however the skin can cause problems for some people including those with IBS, diverticulitis, or other bowel complaints. If this is the case, grill the bell pepper skin side up until blackened, cool, and remove the skins. This also sweetens the taste and you can then marinate them and keep them in the refrigerator for a couple of weeks.

DARK GREEN LEAFY VEGETABLES

Another cliché — "eat your greens"! Well, Mom was right again. Dark green leafy vegetables are 5-star foods and the greener the better. While all leaves provide some nutritional value, the dark green leaves found on the likes of kale, chard, Asian greens, watercress, arugula, spinach, endive, and beet greens are especially good. They are packed with nutrients and phytochemicals thought to play essential roles in our health and well-being, including:

- **FOLATE** — a B vitamin important in fighting cancer and heart disease. Low blood folate levels have been associated with an increased risk of heart disease. Since folate is also essential for cell development and DNA replication, a high folate intake prior to conception and in the first three months of pregnancy has been shown to reduce the incidence of birth defects. Endive, spinach, and savoy cabbage are particularly good sources.

- **LUTEIN AND ZEAXANTHIN** — belong to the carotenoid family of antioxidants and research suggests they are important in keeping your eyes healthy by preventing macular degeneration and possibly cataracts. Kale is an especially abundant source, while spinach, chard, and watercress follow closely behind.

Beware of beta-carotene supplements. A clinical trial had to be stopped after lung cancer incidence actually increased in male smokers and workers exposed to asbestos who were given a supplement containing beta-carotene and vitamin A in combination (Omenn et al, 1996).

- **BETA-CAROTENE** — the most famous carotenoid which gained notoriety from trials linking a high intake to cancer prevention. A similar result was reported from a Finnish trial where again beta-carotene supplements proved detrimental in certain groups, which is more evidence that taking a pill does not have the same effect as consuming a plant-rich diet (The a-tocopherol b-Carotene Cancer Prevention Study Group, 1994). This carotenoid can also be converted to vitamin A in the body when needed, where it then plays an essential role in maintaining good eyesight. Kale again is top here, but spinach, chard, and all dark greens are not far behind.

- **VITAMIN K** — a key vitamin in maintaining healthy blood. Kale, watercress, and chard are especially good sources, but all dark green leafy vegetables provide good amounts of this vitamin.

GLOBE ARTICHOKES

Artichokes have been used since ancient times for various medicinal purposes, including as a treatment for the liver, and there may be a good reason for that — the presence of cynarin (see below). We have to confess that we had almost forgotten this vegetable given that you rarely see it served fresh; it's usually canned or marinated and used in pasta dishes, salads, or as a pizza topping. But we discovered that both the leaves and heart of the artichoke have enormous antioxidant capacity and we had to rethink its dietary value. Cooking with fresh artichokes takes some effort but it's worth a try as they are delicious and it is the most nutritious way to eat them. Canned artichoke hearts are more convenient and certainly good to have in the pantry, but you do miss out on the many phytonutrients found in the leaves. Key nutrients include:

- **CYNARIN** — may prevent fat accumulation in the liver and may also promote the production of bile acids required in digestion.

- **THE FLAVONOID LUTEOLIN** — an antioxidant which seems to be particularly important in preventing damage to LDL-cholesterol, which in turn is involved in the pathogenesis of heart disease. Luteolin may also reduce histamine production and therefore may help reduce the inflammation and congestion associated with hay fever and other allergic reactions.

- **FOLATE** — a B-group vitamin that we now know is important when you are planning a baby, but is also crucial in preventing cancer and heart disease.

MUSHROOMS

Mushrooms are thought of as vegetables, but they are actually a fungus with no roots, leaves, flowers, or seeds. There are many different varieties and each has a slightly different nutrient profile. Most are a good source of the mineral selenium, often low in modern diets. Selenium has an important antioxidant role and is essential for normal functioning of the thyroid gland. They are also fiber rich and, depending on the variety, are good sources of phosphorus, potassium, copper, manganese, and B-group vitamins, including folate.

While even the most common forms of mushrooms have many nutritional benefits, it is worth looking for the more unusual varieties such as the Asian mushrooms, including shiitake, enoki, and maitake, and the large portobello or flat mushrooms. These have higher levels of particular phytonutrients that may benefit our health. Shiitake mushrooms originated in Asia where they have been consumed and used medicinally for thousands of years. Some of the earliest books on Asian herbal medicine discuss the therapeutic value of the shiitake mushroom. Today, scientific research is uncovering various phytochemicals in shiitakes and other mushrooms that may account for the legendary health benefits. These include:

- **LENTINAN** — a polysaccharide shown to have anti-cancer properties in the laboratory. Ongoing studies use extracted lentinan with promising results in cancer patients. It also seems to play a role in strengthening the immune system and early studies indicate it may be of value in the treatment of individuals infected with HIV.

- **ERITADENINE** — a compound shown in studies to lower cholesterol in animals.

- **ERGOTHIONEINE** — a powerful antioxidant found in the highest quantities in mushrooms. Wheat germ and chicken liver were previously thought to be the best sources until mushrooms were tested. Shiitake, oyster, king oyster, and maitake mushrooms were found to contain as much as 40 times the amount found in wheat germ. The more common button mushrooms can't quite match this, but still contain appreciable amounts and up to 12 times as much as that found in wheat germ (Dubost et al, 2005).

As mushrooms are very porous, it is best not to wash them in water; simply wipe them clean with a damp paper towel. Buy them in a paper bag rather than plastic (this makes them sweat and they will quickly become soggy) and store them in the refrigerator for up to a week. You can also buy mushrooms dried for convenience and most of the nutrients will remain intact. Store these in an airtight container in the refrigerator or freezer where they will stay fresh for as long as a year.

THE ONION FAMILY

The onion family, technically called the *Alliums*, includes not only onions but also leeks, garlic, shallots, and green onions. These vegetables seem to be particularly important in preventing cancer of the stomach, but also play a healthy role throughout the gut and in lowering the risk of cardiovascular disease. Unfortunately, cooking at high heat destroys some of the disease-fighting nutrients, particularly diallyl sulfide, and we often start a dish by frying the garlic and onion. You might want to try adding them later to a dish or eating them raw on occasion to maximize the health benefits. You may find that raw garlic is not so easy on your digestion; if so, removing the small green shoot from the middle of the clove before eating sometimes does the trick.

Some of the key nutrients found in these 5-star vegetables are:

- **SULPHUR COMPOUNDS** — including diallyl sulfide, are shown in research to prevent tumor growth in the stomach, colon, and liver. Onions and garlic are particularly good sources.

- **ANTIOXIDANTS** — leeks contain kaempferol, which is a flavonoid, red onions have quercetin, and don't throw away the green tops of leeks and green onions as these contain the antioxidant carotenoids lutein and zeaxanthin. Both are important for eye health and reduce the risk of age-related macular degeneration and cataracts.

- **GARLIC** — has antibacterial qualities and this may be of benefit in destroying potential harmful bacteria in food and in our stomach.

- **FRUCTO-OLIGOSACCHARIDES (FOS)** — you have no doubt heard of probiotics (where you consume live beneficial bacteria), but these compounds are prebiotics. They act like fiber in that they pass through the small intestine undigested and enter the colon. There they feed the beneficial bacteria already present, promoting their growth. The byproducts of this bacterial fermentation benefit us in many ways including keeping stool soft and easy to pass, keeping the cells lining the colon healthy (preventing cancers), and boosting immune function.

PARSLEY — FLAT-LEAF AND CURLY

You might think of parsley as simply a garnish to make a bowl of soup look nice, but that would be to grossly underestimate the herb's nutritional value. Parsley is packed with nutrients including vitamin K, involved primarily in blood clotting, vitamin C, several B-group vitamins, useful amounts of iron and other minerals, and the carotenoids beta-carotene, lutein, and zeaxanthin. Beta-carotene is an important antioxidant in its own right, helping to protect the fat-soluble areas of the body, but can also be converted to vitamin A when required. Both lutein and zeaxanthin have been associated with a reduction in the risk of age-related macular degeneration of the eye, a common cause of blindness, and lutein has additionally been shown to play a possible role in preventing colon cancer. Of course, one sprig won't do much good; you need to use more of it to gain the benefits. The classic Middle Eastern dish tabouli is packed with fresh parsley, or you could liberally add it at the end of cooking to sauces, soups, casseroles, or mix it in a salad.

PEAS — GREEN AND SUGAR SNAP/SNOW PEAS

For peas we include green peas (fresh or frozen) and sugar snap/snow peas, which are just a variety of peas that we eat pod and all. All varieties of peas contain a wealth of important nutrients including the carotenoids beta-carotene, alpha-carotene, lutein, and zeaxanthin. While all of these have the potential to act as powerful disease-fighting antioxidants, they are also important for eye health. In the body, alpha- and beta-carotene can be converted to vitamin A, a nutrient essential for good vision, while lutein and zeaxanthin are found in abundance in the eye and reduce the risk of age-related macular degeneration. Green peas are particularly rich in lutein and zeaxanthin. All peas are fiber rich and therefore great for your digestive tract. As with other legumes, they are high in soluble fiber that binds to cholesterol in the stomach, helping to reduce blood levels. Peas also provide a range of vitamins and minerals — in particular, the antioxidant vitamin C, vitamin K, required for healthy blood and strong bones, the B-group vitamins necessary for carbohydrate, protein, and fat metabolism, and iron for normal blood cell formation and function. Peas do provide a higher carbohydrate level than other vegetables, and therefore slightly more calories but, given that you are highly unlikely to overeat them, this is really not a concern! They also provide a reasonable amount of plant protein and so are a particularly good inclusion in vegetarian diets.

TOMATOES

We hear lots about the antioxidants vitamins A, C, and E and beta-carotene, but we hope you are getting the picture that there are in fact many more antioxidants found in food. Tomatoes are listed among our top veggies because they contain lycopene, an antioxidant that may be even more powerful than vitamin C. Lycopene is found in other red foods, such as pink grapefruit and watermelon, but undoubtedly the best sources are tomatoes and tomato products. In fact, this is an unusual case where food processing actually increases the availability of the nutrient, as shown below.

LYCOPENE IN FOODS

PRODUCT	LYCOPENE (milligrams/ 100 grams)	SERVING SIZE	LYCOPENE (milligrams/ serving)
Tomato paste	42.2	2 tablespoons	13.8
Pasta sauce	21.9	½ cup	28.1
Tomato sauce (ketchup)	14.1	¼ cup	8.9
Tomato juice	9.5	1 cup	25.0
Pink grapefruit	4.0	½ fruit	4.9
Raw tomato	3.0	1 medium	3.7

From the table above, you can see that tomato paste is fabulously rich in lycopene, especially when compared to a raw tomato. Try adding tomato paste into soups, sauces, and casseroles; add a dash of Worcestershire sauce and Tabasco to tomato juice for a spicy refreshing drink; or try our recipe for Basic Tomato and Basil Sauce on page 197. While there is no consensus yet on how much we need, the best studies from Harvard (Giovannucci 1999) suggest we should be eating one or two tomato products every day.

But, it's not all about lycopene, other goodies in tomatoes include:

- **BETA-CAROTENE** — a potent antioxidant linked to reduced cancer risk when consumed in foods (infamously not so when consumed as a supplement where it can actually increase cancer growth rate, see page 16 under dark green leafy vegetables).

- **CAFFEIC AND FERULIC ACIDS** — involved in the production of cancer-fighting enzymes in the body.

- **CHLOROGENIC ACID** — believed to help detoxify carcinogens and viruses.

- **LUTEIN AND ZEAXANTHIN** — the carotenoids we have met several times already, thought to be important in preventing eye disease.

World's Healthiest Fruits ✩ ✩ ✩ ✩ ✩

APRICOTS, FRESH AND DRIED

The wonderful orange color in apricots comes from the carotenoids present in them. They are particularly high in the potent antioxidant beta-carotene. Only three apricots provide about half of the daily amount of beta-carotene experts recommend. Beta-carotene is believed to play a role in preventing damage to cells from free radicals that lead to heart disease, cancer, and accelerated aging. It can also be converted to vitamin A, essential for good vision, when intakes of this vitamin are insufficient. Fresh apricots are also good sources of vitamin C, adding to the antioxidant power of the fruit as well as being essential for a strong immune function and healthy skin. Drying the fruit unfortunately destroys much of the vitamin C, but most of the other nutrients are preserved and are, indeed, concentrated in this form. Dried apricots of course have a higher energy density so if you are watching your weight you can't eat unlimited amounts. However, they do have a low GI and make a great between-meal snack. The dried fruit is a particularly good source of iron, essential for the production of properly functioning red blood cells, and is also a good laxative.

AVOCADOS

The days of the low-fat dogma have cast a shadow on the poor avocado, yet it has so much to offer us. Yes, it does indeed contain a lot of fat, so you can't eat it until the cows come home, but you are unlikely to given its rich flavor. The fat in avocados is predominately unsaturated, and mostly monounsaturated like that found in olive oil. This makes it an ideal replacement for butter on bread, and you can buy avocado oil for cooking and to use in salad dressings. This type of fat not only benefits our cholesterol levels and in reduces cardiovascular disease risk, but it also seems to be more easily burned as fuel rather than being deposited on our hips — all good news if you are battling with weight control. Not only that, but avocados also give us:

Preservatives such as sulphites are often used in the processing of dried fruits. Those with asthma, especially children, may be particularly sensitive and should avoid this preservative. Look for preservative-free or organic produce to avoid this.

- **VITAMIN E** — the major fat-soluble antioxidant that protects the fatty outer layers of cells from free-radical damage.

- **VITAMIN C** — a water-soluble antioxidant that strengthens the immune system, and also recycles vitamin E, keeping it functioning. This is an example of how no nutrient works in isolation but in partnership with others.

- **FOLATE** — essential for women planning a baby, but also in preventing heart disease by lowering homocysteine levels in the blood, and in reducing the risk of cancer, as folate is key in the production of DNA and new cells.

- **FIBER** — half an avocado provides 6–7 grams of fiber, putting you well on your way to meeting your daily target of 25–30 grams.

- **VITAMIN K** — plays an essential role in blood clotting.

- **GLUTATHIONE** — an antioxidant involved in preventing free-radical damage to cells.

- **POTASSIUM AND MAGNESIUM** — both may help keep blood pressure down. Magnesium can also help migraine sufferers and reduce symptoms of PMS.

- **BETA-SITOSTEROL** — a compound currently being studied for its potential to prevent breast cancer. It may also reduce the symptoms of prostate enlargement (benign prostatic hyperplasia or BPH) that often plagues men as they get older.

BERRIES

Berries look and taste delicious, so it seems too good to be true that they are actually good for us. Yet berries are tops when it comes to comparing the antioxidant power of all plant foods, and they are packed with other nutrients our bodies need.

Key nutrients found in berries include:

- **ANTHOCYANINS** — a subgroup of the flavonoids and responsible for the purple/red color of berries; these are powerful antioxidant compounds.

- **ELLAGIC ACID** — particularly rich in strawberries, raspberries, and blackberries and seems to have anti-cancer properties. In laboratory experiments it has been shown to induce cancer-cell death and act as an antioxidant (Han et al, 2006).

- **KAEMPFEROL** — yet another antioxidant which may also reduce LDL-cholesterol.

- **TANNINS** — found in cranberries, blackberries, and blueberries; can prevent bacteria from attaching to the urinary tract and thus are useful in staving off cystitis.

- **VITAMIN C** — is important in maintaining a strong immune system and is essential in the production of collagen. Healthy skin therefore relies on a good vitamin C intake. Strawberries and fresh cranberries are particularly rich in it.

CANTALOUPE

Cantaloupe is wonderfully rich in vitamin C and its orange color comes from the carotenoids present in it. It is particularly rich in beta-carotene, containing more than other types of melon. Beta-carotene from foods has been linked to the prevention of cancers and heart disease (taking the antioxidant as a supplement may, rather alarmingly, have the opposite effect, see page 16 under dark green leafy vegetables). The body can also convert it to vitamin A, essential for good vision. Since vitamin A is primarily found in animal fat such as full-fat dairy foods and butter, this can be a good way to ensure you meet vitamin A requirements while reducing your intake of these foods.

Cantaloupe is also high in potassium, important in reducing blood pressure, and the soluble fiber pectin, useful in reducing blood cholesterol. Cantaloupe may, therefore, help to reduce the risk of heart disease and stroke.

CITRUS FRUIT

Unfortunately, for many people, drinking orange juice is the closest they come to enjoying the benefits of citrus fruit. This group includes oranges of all varieties, tangerines, mandarins, clementines, grapefruit, pink grapefruit, lemons, and limes. Vitamin C probably comes to mind as the key nutrient and, indeed, a single orange provides about one-and-a-half times your daily requirement (and we suspect more may be beneficial). Many of us reach for vitamin C supplements when we have a cold or flu and we may be right to do so. A recent review of the evidence concluded that, while vitamin C does not seem to stop you from catching the cold, it is indeed involved in respiratory defenses and has an (albeit small) benefit in reducing the duration and severity of the infection (Douglas et al, 2004). Our advice is to forget the supplements and tuck into the real thing instead; you'll certainly do no harm this way and just might do much good.

Besides, it's not all about vitamin C. Here are just some of the beneficial nutrients and phytochemicals to be found in these wonderful fruits:

- **FIBER** — contributes to citrus's low GI in part due to its good amounts of the soluble fiber pectin, which slows the absorption of the carbohydrates. The pith also contains insoluble fiber which acts like a broom sweeping through the intestines, keeping you regular and your digestion healthy.

- **FOLATE** — an essential B-group vitamin that can prevent neural tube defects in newborns, reduce your risk of heart disease and fight cancer by keeping new cell development healthy.

> Frozen fruit is usually just as nutritious as fresh — sometimes more so as nutrients easily lost in storage or with exposure to light, such as vitamin C, are preserved. Furthermore, freezing is itself a preservative meaning that artificial preservatives need not be added.

- **LIMONENE AND COUMARIN** — found in the skin, these are antioxidants which have been shown to stimulate a detoxification enzyme that in turn protects tissues from free-radical damage. Don't worry, we're not going to suggest you start eating the skin of your orange, but using the zest in dishes is a good plan to make sure you reap all the benefits from these fruits.

- **BETA-CRYPTOXANTHIN** — another of the carotenoid group of antioxidants, found particularly in orange fruits. Studies are investigating its role in the prevention of colon cancer.

- **NARINGIN** — a flavonoid antioxidant found in grapefruit, and has a role in protecting the lungs from toxins in the air from pollution and cigarette smoke (as does vitamin C).

- **NOBILETIN** — another flavonoid found in the flesh of oranges, and is shown to have anti-inflammatory properties.

- **TANGERETIN** — yet another flavonoid, this time found in mandarins, is being studied for its potential to reduce tumor growth.

GUAVAS

We tend to think of citrus fruits as being the best source of vitamin C when in fact guavas top them all. One fruit provides more than double your vitamin C requirements for the day. Guavas are also rich in carotenoids, particularly lycopene, which is more often associated with tomatoes. There is some evidence to show that a high lycopene intake reduces the risk of cardiovascular disease, certain cancers including prostate cancer, and perhaps macular degenerative disease. The fiber in guavas is great for digestion and can help to reduce cholesterol levels and the fruit is also a good source of folate, potassium, copper, and manganese.

KIWIFRUIT

This strange-looking, hairy fruit (who on earth first thought it might be good to eat?) is one of the richest dietary sources of vitamin C. Just one kiwifruit provides roughly double the recommended daily intake. Aside from the roles already mentioned, vitamin C also enhances our absorption of non-animal source iron. It is therefore a good idea to slice a kiwifruit on your muesli or breakfast cereal in the morning, or to finish a vegetarian meal with the fruit. A few other goodies to be found below the fuzzy skin are:

- LUTEIN — one of the carotenoids important for eye health and may also be important in preventing colon cancer.

- CHLOROGENIC ACID — an antioxidant which seems to play a role in preventing tumor growth.

- FIBER — has benefits for the digestive tract and also ensures that the fruit sugars are absorbed slowly, minimizing the impact on blood sugar.

MANGOES

One of the wonderful things about the start of summer is that mangoes come into season. These delicious tropical fruits are a real treat both in taste and nutrition. They provide several nutrients including vitamin C, vitamin B6, and fiber. Mangoes are also incredibly rich in beta-carotene, much richer than other fruits, hence their wonderful orange color. This alone credits the mango as a 5-star food. Enjoy them sliced on your muesli for breakfast, chopped in a salsa, and served with chicken, or try the Avocado, Mango, and Pine Nut Salad (page 186).

PAPAYAS

The orange color in papaya comes from the presence of carotenoids, which are present in a wide range of varieties. The fruit is a particularly good source of beta-crytoxanthin, which has been shown in studies to reduce the risk of lung and colon cancers. Other studies have linked this antioxidant to a reduction in the risk of rheumatoid arthritis — a condition also caused in part by free-radical damage. Papaya is also rich in vitamin C and the fiber is useful in maintaining healthy digestion and low blood cholesterol. We find the taste of papaya is much improved by squeezing the juice of a lime over the cut fruit.

PASSION FRUIT

Passion fruit are packed with fiber, providing more than double the amount in the same weight of most other fruits. Aside from benefiting your digestive tract, the presence of soluble fiber can help to reduce blood cholesterol. They are also full of vitamin C and contain good levels of pro-vitamin A carotenoids. The good levels of potassium can help to lower blood pressure.

PERSIMMONS

Persimmons are not among the most well-known fruits, but we urge you to be adventurous and try them if you haven't already done so. The rich color comes from the carotenoids and persimmons are particularly rich in beta-crytoxanthin. This carotenoid has been linked in studies to a reduced risk of colon cancer, lung cancer, and rheumatoid arthritis. They are also good sources of fiber (twice as much as an apple), potassium, magnesium, manganese, and even provide the minerals calcium and iron in useful quantities.

There are two types of the fruit commonly available — the Hachiya persimmon should be eaten when completely ripe and soft, while the Fuyu is smaller and eaten when firm and crisp like an apple. You can eat them raw, mash them up to use in muffins, toss them into a green salad, or cook the flesh in a little olive oil, blend it, and use it as a glaze for chicken or meat.

POMEGRANATES

Pomegranates may never have made it to your fruit bowl, probably because many of us don't know what to do with them. That's a shame because they are hard to beat for antioxidant power. If you have never tried one you are in for a treat — both in taste and in nutritional benefit. The word pomegranate actually means "seeded apple" and this is essentially what it is. The round, crimson fruit is packed with clusters of seeds of the same wonderful color. Pomegranates are rich in vitamin C, fiber, and three different types of polyphenols credited with helping in the prevention of heart disease and cancer:

- TANNINS — also found in tea and red wine, and responsible for the slightly astringent or bitter taste in these foods. Tannins are better known for their negative effect in binding minerals such as iron, and reducing their absorption. However, in plants, tannins have powerful antimicrobial and antioxidant properties. This has stimulated research into whether these same positive attributes apply when eaten rather than drunk.

- **ANTHOCYANINS** — a subgroup of the flavonoids, and responsible for the purple/red color of pomegranates; these are powerful antioxidant compounds.

- **ELLAGIC ACID** — seems to have anti-cancer properties. In laboratory experiments it has been shown to induce cancer-cell death and act as an antioxidant.

Pomegranate juice has hit the shelves in a big way with companies promoting its antioxidant content. While the juice does indeed provide these powerful antioxidants, just watch out for any added sugar. Read the ingredients list to be sure of what else you are getting. As with all fruit juices, pomegranate juice is certainly nutrient rich but also calorie rich — which won't help your waistline. It is almost always better to eat the whole fruit.

Pomegranates are not difficult to prepare when you know how. Try this easy method recommended by the Pomegranate Council in California (www. pomegranates.org) — they call it 3 Step-No Mess!

1. Cut off the crown and cut the pomegranate into sections.

2. Place the sections in a bowl of water, then roll out the arils (juice sacs) with your fingers. Discard everything else.

3. Strain out the water then eat the succulent arils whole, seeds and all.

PRUNES

Famous for their ability to promote regularity, prunes are simply dried plums. More energy dense than the fresh fruit, they are very nutritious — many of their nutrients survive the drying process and are then concentrated in the prune. Promoting healthy bacterial fermentation and good digestive health, their high-fiber content adds bulk to intestinal contents, promoting movement through the gut and fueling the bacteria present in the colon. Prunes also have real antioxidant power — they contain different phenols that help to protect the fat-soluble areas of the body from free-radical damage. Their very low GI makes them an ideal snack.

CARBOHYDRATES

WORLD'S HEALTHIEST CARBOHYDRATES

☆ ☆ ☆ ☆ ☆

Barley — Pot and Pearl

Beans and Lentils (including red kidney beans, black-eyed peas, lima beans, green beans, chickpeas, canellini beans, butter beans, mung beans, and all lentils)

Breads (including grainy sourdough, pumpernickel, traditional stoneground, and whole grain)

Buckwheat

Bulgur

Corn

Freekeh

Oats and Natural Mueseli

Quinoa

Whole-Grain Pasta

They're in and then they're out. Poor old carbohydrates have taken quite a beating over recent years as diet after diet hits the shelves blaming these foods for expanding waistlines and almost every chronic disease plaguing the Western world. Yet, health authorities and most dietitians continue to promote a high-carbohydrate diet as the healthy choice. It's little wonder so many people are completely confused about whose advice to follow.

There are elements of truth on both sides of the argument, and that is because you cannot simply lump all carbohydrate-rich foods in one basket and say carbs are good or bad. We have to consider the qualities of the individual food before we say if it is a good or bad choice. So what would make a carb a good choice? Take a look at the following chart.

THE BEST CARBS WILL	THE WORST CARBS WILL
fill us up and keep us satisfied between meals so that we eat less and don't snack on the wrong things	be rapidly digested and absorbed leading to glucose "spikes" in the blood after eating, which damages blood vessels
deliver glucose slowly and steadily into the blood, keeping our blood sugar steady	lead to a rapid fall in blood glucose an hour or two after eating, stimulating hunger and inducing cravings, especially for sweet foods
be rich in different types of fiber to keep us regular, keep our bowels healthy, and keep our cholesterol down	stimulate a big release of insulin which, if frequent, will increase fat storage, reduce fat burning, and become a risk factor for heart disease
be nutritionally rich, providing an array of vitamins, minerals, and phytochemicals such as antioxidants	provide carbohydrates but little else — "empty calories"
reduce our risk of chronic disease including heart disease, type 2 diabetes, and certain cancers	increase our risk of chronic disease including heart disease, type 2 diabetes, and certain cancers

Looking at carbs in this way makes it easy to see why there is so much controversy, and it also makes it easy to see how we can reap the benefits without the pitfalls. The best choices are obviously those that deliver as many of these attributes as possible. The clear winners are vegetables, fruits, whole grains, and legumes. These are the least common choices in most Western diets and it is therefore not surprising that carbs have been blamed for many of our ills. Vegetables and fruits are so important and absolutely essential in any healthy diet, that we have categorized them all on their own. So in this section we will focus on the bigger sources of carbohydrates in our diet — for most people that means bread, pasta, rice, breakfast cereal, cakes, cookies, other grains, and legumes. We'll introduce you to a few you may never have tried, or may never even have heard of, and we'll no doubt disappoint you by relegating a few of your favorites to the 1-star category, but by making better choices more often you have the potential to dramatically change the way you look, feel, and live.

WHY DO WE NEED CARBS?

There are many good reasons to include carbohydrates in your healthy eating menu, including:

- for optimal cognitive performance
- to perform at our best during exercise
- to maintain a healthy bowel
- carbs are relatively cheap, readily available, and easy to store.

FOR OPTIMAL COGNITIVE PERFORMANCE

Our brain (and certain other cells in the body including red blood cells) runs almost exclusively on glucose — the carbohydrate that circulates in our blood. While we can make glucose from protein, there is a limit to our rate and capacity to do so. For our bodies to function, blood glucose must not fall below a certain level. If it were to drop dangerously low, we would fall into a coma and, without intervention, could die. That is why our bodies can make glucose from protein: It is a fall-back system to ensure there is a constant glucose supply for the brain. In times of famine, the brain adapts and can run on ketone bodies made from fat, but this is not normal metabolism and certainly not the preferred fuel. Since carbohydrates are clearly an essential fuel in our bodies, it makes sense to bring in fuel in the form it is needed. Research shows that brain function — including memory and concentration — is much improved after eating carbohydrate-containing foods, particularly first thing in the morning. You may have experienced this yourself if you have tried following a low-carbohydrate diet — common complaints are of headaches, lack of concentration, and poor memory.

TO PERFORM AT OUR BEST DURING EXERCISE

When we exercise, glucose and fat are used as fuel, but glucose becomes increasingly important as the intensity of the exercise increases. Think of fat as the tortoise — the slow steady burner that can run for a long time but cannot go very fast. Glucose, on the other hand, is the hare — it can produce a lot of energy fast but without refueling will run out pretty quickly. Because we cannot turn protein into glucose quickly enough during exercise, we need to have a good store of glucose ready before we start and to adequately fill these glucose stores we need to eat carbohydrate-containing food.

Making exercise a regular part of your life is not an optional extra — it is essential if you want to look, feel, and perform at your best. This means that you will need to eat sufficient carbs to support your exercise program. Of course, this also means that the more you exercise the more carbs you need and vice versa; but remember, not exercising and not eating carbs means you miss out on the irreplaceable benefits of both.

TO MAINTAIN A HEALTHY BOWEL

It's interesting that constipation is almost unheard of in native cultures yet is one of the most common complaints in the Western world. Chronic constipation can lead to all sorts of problems including bloating, digestion, abdominal pain, flatulence, hemorrhoids, diverticulitis, and bowel cancer. Our sedentary lifestyle plays a huge part in this. An inactive body leads to an inactive gut. A key dietary difference is the amount of fiber we consume.

Fiber is, in fact, just carbohydrate, but of a type that we cannot break down and absorb in the small intestine. Therefore, it comes as no surprise to discover the best sources of fiber are also carb-rich foods. If you choose to follow a low-carb diet you inevitably end up with a low-fiber diet and your bowel will suffer as a result.

Fiber acts like a broom through the digestive system — it absorbs water to swell the intestine's contents, which in turn stimulates the intestinal walls to contract and sweep the contents along. Once it reaches the large intestine or colon it is fermented by the resident bacteria-producing substances that feed the cells of the colon and keep them healthy. Water is reabsorbed here and waste matter is eliminated. Modern diets with little fiber contain far more digestible and readily absorbed food. This sounds good but actually means that by the time the stomach contents have reached the colon there is little left and it moves slowly. More and more water is absorbed, making the content drier, more compact, and ... you get the picture. This means that waste products and potentially carcinogenic compounds hang around longer in the colon where they can do their damage. Gas builds up, adding to the problem, and you are left feeling bloated, blocked up, and sluggish. To avoid this, you need both fiber and enough water in your diet to keep the fiber-rich intestinal contents fluid.

There are many types of fiber but they are generally classified as insoluble or soluble. Insoluble fiber is mostly found in the outer husk of a grain — the bran. This is removed when grains are polished (for example, in white rice) or processed (for example, to produce white flour). Insoluble fiber is also found in the fibrous parts of vegetables and the skin of legumes and some fruits. This type of fiber is best for keeping you regular and preventing constipation.

The other major type of fiber is soluble fiber. As the name suggests, this type of fiber is (at least partly) soluble in water and forms a sort of gel in the stomach. Soluble fiber is particularly beneficial in two ways. It can "trap" cholesterol in the stomach — both the cholesterol in bile salts secreted by the liver and the cholesterol in the foods we eat — and prevent it from being absorbed. This has a small but clinically important effect in lowering blood cholesterol levels. It is for this reason that oats, a grain rich in this type of fiber, are often cited as a good cholesterol-lowering food. Secondly, the gel-like formation slows down the access of digestive enzymes to the carbohydrate present in the gut contents, which in turn slows the absorption of that carbohydrate into the bloodstream. Soluble fiber is therefore intrinsically linked to the GI of the food — foods high in soluble fiber invariably have a low GI. Legumes are a good example of this and one of the reasons they warrant 5-star status.

CARBS ARE RELATIVELY CHEAP, READILY AVAILABLE, AND EASY TO STORE

From a purely practical point of view, cutting out carbs makes life very difficult, not to mention unsociable. Carbs are relatively cheap, you can store them in the pantry, making it easier to put together a healthy home-cooked meal without shopping every day, and they are widely available: Even your local corner shop will stock bread at the very least. The same cannot be said of fresh protein-rich foods.

PROCESSED HIGH FIBER VS. NATURALLY HIGH IN FIBER

Many packaged foods labeled "high fiber" are not the best choice. Many are simply heavily processed grain foods or have a whole host of other added ingredients, with some bran fiber thrown in to disguise it as a healthy product. Granola bars are a good example — yes, they contain oats and can boast a good amount of fiber, but many also have added hydrogenated fats, syrups, and refined sugars which bump up their calorie and unhealthy fat content. Many high-fiber breakfast cereals are processed cereals with bran fiber added back in. While they are certainly a better choice than low-fiber cereals, the majority have a high GI since the fiber added is insoluble and does not slow the digestive enzymes.

In fact, there is a major problem with eating too much of this type of insoluble cereal fiber. It contains compounds called phytates which bind to minerals including iron, zinc, and calcium, preventing them from being absorbed by the body. Too much cereal fiber can therefore leave you deficient in one or more of these minerals. The ubiquitous scattering of bran fiber in particular into many of our so-called healthy foods is a double-edged sword — it might be helping our digestion, but in those who diligently choose the high-fiber option too often they may be doing more harm than good.

The solution is to choose foods naturally high in fiber rather than too many foods with fiber added. You will then benefit from both the fiber as well as the full array of nutrients that food has to offer. A variety of our 5-star carbs will fit the bill nicely.

The GI — an invaluable tool for choosing quality carbs

Proponents of high-protein/low-carbohydrate diets argue that grains have made us fat. The major flaw in this argument is that we have eaten grains for thousands of years, yet have really only become fat in the last 50. In fact, much of the exponential rise in obesity has been in the last 20 years. Genetic susceptibility undoubtedly plays a part but cannot explain the full story. We have to ask: What has changed in the last few decades to make us so prone to getting fat?

WHAT DO WE DO TO THE GRAIN?

When humans started to eat grain foods, we harvested the grain and roughly ground it between stones to crack the hard outer shell, added water to the resultant mix, and then cooked it in some way. Over time, we learned how to use grain to make bread, cook porridge, or add it to thicken stews. We learned that grains could bulk up a meal, making the meat go a lot further while filling everyone up relatively cheaply.

It's the same story today — animal foods tend to be much more expensive while grain foods are cheap and readily available. But we have now learned how to grind the grain, remove the tough outer husk, and polish the grain down to just the starch-rich center. We can then cook the polished grain to make a fluffy white rice, for example, or can grind this starch center to a fine flour to produce fluffy white breads. Or we take the fine flour and mix it with fat and/or sugar and make cookies, cakes, crackers, breakfast cereals, and so on. You can see that over time, with sophisticated food-manufacturing techniques, we have moved further and further away from the grain in its natural state. In fact, all we do is strip the grain of almost all its fiber and micronutrient content, and use only the energy-containing part of the grain — the starchy center. The real change in the last 50 years has been in what we do to the grains in our diet.

HOW DOES THIS PROCESSING AFFECT THE BODY?

We can measure the effect of this processing on our body and see the physiological change quite clearly. When carbohydrate-containing foods are eaten, the food is digested and broken down in the intestines to release the individual sugars, principally glucose. These sugars are then absorbed into the bloodstream where the glucose is transported to cells all around the body to be used as fuel or stored for later use. How quickly this happens varies depending on the food. This is the basis for the glycemic index or GI. The GI compares foods, gram for gram, of carbohydrates by directly measuring the rise in blood glucose after eating the food.

In the GI, the response to pure glucose is called 100 and all other foods are compared and ranked accordingly. High-GI foods have values of 70 or more (in other words they produce a response equal to or greater than 70 percent that of pure glucose), moderate-GI foods have values in the range 56 to 69, and low-GI foods have values of 55 or less (in other words, they produce a response of 55 percent or less that of pure glucose).

If we directly compare the GI of grains under increasing levels of processing — whole grains, cracked grains, whole-wheat flour and so on to refined flour — we see a stepped increase in the glycemic response. Compared to the diets of our ancestors, it is clear that the glycemic impact today is far greater since we eat more high-GI foods. In other words, the rises and falls in our blood glucose levels today are larger than in the past.

Our bodies are just not designed to deal with these rapid and large fluctuations in blood glucose. Glucose levels in the blood need to stay fairly stable and there are systems in place to do just that. When glucose levels rise in the blood after eating carbohydrates, the pancreas releases the hormone insulin. Insulin acts like a key allowing glucose entry into cells around the body. For example, muscle cells take up glucose to use as fuel, or they can store the glucose for later use; the brain needs a constant supply of glucose; and the liver also stores some glucose that it can release between meals to prevent blood levels from falling too low. This system works beautifully when there is the right amount of glucose coming in from the digestive tract, the right amount of insulin being released, and the right amount of glucose being used up by active muscles. Problems start when the system is overloaded, overworked, or malfunctioning.

Overloading happens when you eat a large amount of carbohydrates all at once, and/or eat carbohydrates that are rapidly absorbed, like high-GI foods. A modern breakfast consisting of a large bowl of cornflakes followed by white bread toast will result in overload for most people. The system becomes overworked when this happens on a regular basis where modern diets are filled with high-carbohydrate, high-GI foods. The system malfunctions when not enough insulin is produced to do the job, or when the insulin produced does not work effectively. This happens in those with insulin resistance and diabetes. In the U.S. it is estimated that 8 percent of the population has diabetes and that 24 percent of those people don't know it (American Diabetes Association). They are a ticking time bomb with increased risk of heart disease and related conditions. The body also malfunctions when we are too sedentary — inactive lifestyles cause us to lose muscle and this increases our risk of developing insulin resistance which can lead to diabetes.

Are you at risk of having insulin resistance? A good indicator is the size of your waist. Regardless of your height, your waist circumference tells you how much fat you have stored around your middle. It is this fat that is most problematic and one of the causes of insulin resistance. Get a tape measure and, without clothing, measure around your middle. For men and some women, directly around the navel is a good guide; for "hourglass-shaped" women, choose the narrowest point. For men, a measurement of less than 37 inches is healthy; 37–40 inches shows an increased risk of insulin resistance; and more than 40 inches shows a great risk. For women, a measurement of less than 31.5 inches is healthy; 31.5–34.5 inches shows an increased risk of insulin resistance; and more than 34.5 inches shows a great risk. (Note: These cut-offs apply to those with Caucasian heritage. If you are of Pacific Island origin, you can add 4 inches to these cut-offs, but if of Asian origin you need to subtract 4 inches.)

Glucose "spikes" after eating high-GI meals have been shown to damage blood vessels and cause a low level of inflammation around the body. High levels of insulin are also damaging and hyperinsulinemia (high insulin in the blood) is a known risk factor for cardiovascular disease. You can control both of these factors by choosing low, rather than high, GI foods at most meals. The occasional high-GI food will do no harm, so long as your overall diet has a low GI. The vast majority of traditional diets around the world do in fact have a low GI, while the majority of high-GI foods are modern processed grain foods that have entered our diet in the last few decades. This is shown in the table on page 37.

TRADITIONAL LOW GI FOODS	MODERN HIGH GI FOODS
stoneground breads	white bread
sourdough breads	regular whole-wheat bread
heavy, grainy breads	most polished white rice
porridge, oats, and granola	most breakfast cereals
pasta	most cereal snack bars and cookies
legumes (lentils and beans)	potatoes
most fruit	french fries
barley	scones and english muffins
quinoa	bagels
cracked wheat	
buckwheat	
rye	

GI classifications taken from the International Table of Glycemic Index and Glycemic Load Values: 2002 (Foster-Powell et al, 2002) and the online database at www.glycemicindex.com.

The GI can sound very complicated and scientific but there is no need to get bogged down in the theory. Neither is there any need to know the GI of every single food you eat. All you need to consider is the GI of the major sources of carbohydrates in your diet — and we have done the planning for you. All of our 5-star foods, and most of our 4-star foods, have a low GI. Choose these on most occasions and you will achieve a low-GI diet. It's that simple.

LESSONS FROM THE PAST

One way of determining the optimal human diet is to look back in time. What have we evolved eating and can we compare that to what we are eating now? It is not an easy process to determine what man ate hundreds, thousands, and millions of years ago, but scientists have good clues and evidence to work with to give us a fair idea. The best evidence points to the fact that man ate an animal-food-dominated diet in the pre-agricultural age. This is hunter-gatherer man at his iconic best — the men out hunting wild animals, catching fish and seafood, while the women gathered plant foods such as native vegetables and fruits. Animal foods certainly were the major source of energy, but the plant foods provided large quantities of fiber and micronutrients, including antioxidants. Grains would not have been eaten to any large extent at this time, simply because, without modern farming and milling equipment, they would have been too labor intensive.

Then came the agricultural age, so-called because people learned how to farm the land, and grow and harvest crops to support their communities. This happened some 10,000 years ago, and from this time cereal grains became an increasingly important part of human diets around the world. When we look at the entire pathway through history of how we have evolved, this is a small step on a very long road. This is the reason why many believe that, genetically, we have not yet evolved to cope with the change from predominately animal-based to predominately cereal-based foods in our diet (Cordain et al, 2005).

If we step forward in time, today we find that almost every community around the world eats approximately the same percentage of their energy intake from protein; 15–18 percent compared to the estimated 19–35 percent of our hunter-gatherer ancestors (Cordain et al, 2002). The amount of carbohydrates we eat varies across countries, but grains and foods made from whole grain are now major dietary players.

At the same time, rates of obesity and chronic diseases are on the rise and, because of this, many believe that we should return to a diet closer to that of our hunter-gatherer ancestors. This is a valid argument and, for some, achieving such a diet may well be advantageous. But there has been a lot of misinterpretation of what such a diet is. The current fad of low-carbohydrate eating takes on various forms but these are not hunter-gatherer diets. There are some key differences:

1 FRUIT USUALLY BANNED ON A LOW-CARB DIET.

Fruit is almost always cut out or restricted because it contains sugar and therefore is bad, yet what can be more natural than eating something that grows from the land, as the "gatherers" would have done? These same diets will go on to recommend various protein powders and bars, egg replacers, and other processed, manufactured food products. How can this possibly be better for us than eating a carbohydrate-containing banana?

2 VEGETABLES SEVERELY RESTRICTED IN TYPE AND/OR QUANTITY.

Hunter-gatherers ate large quantities of plant foods, including vegetables. In fact, estimates for their fiber intakes are in the range of approximately 90 grams a day, compared to the average of 15 grams a day in Western diets. Diets that restrict vegetables are restricting your fiber and micronutrient intake at the same time.

3 DIFFERENCES IN MEAT FROM DOMESTICATED AND WILD ANIMALS.

Hunter-gatherers ate wild animals, fish, and seafood. Today we mostly eat domesticated animals, and even farmed fish and seafood is becoming the norm. There are key nutritional differences between the two, primarily concerning the type of fat present. Meat from animals in the wild tends to be lower in total and saturated fat and much higher in the fats we know to be good for us, particularly the omega-3 fats. Furthermore, even the type of saturated fat present differs. Saturated fats are classified by their molecular chain length, and not all of these fats raise cholesterol levels. It is the shorter-chain saturated fats that appear to be responsible. These undesirable fats are the predominant saturated fat in meat from domesticated animals. In contrast, the saturated fat present in meat from animals living in their natural habitat, eating their native diet, is predominately one of the longer-chain fats, called stearic acid. This fat does not raise blood cholesterol. This means that a high-animal-produce diet today is nutritionally different to the high-animal-produce diet of our hunter-gatherer ancestors.

4 MODERN HIGH-MEAT DIETS LINKED TO COLON CANCER.

High-meat diets today have been linked to an increased risk of colon cancer (Larsson and Wolk, 2006). The greatest risk comes from eating processed meat products, including burgers and sausages, which would not have been a part of our ancestors' diet, and from eating charred meat. Burning the meat surface produces carcinogens, so be particularly careful as to how you cook meat on the barbecue and avoid overcooked, blackened meat. Hunter-gatherer man may have been protected by the simultaneous consumption of high quantities of fibrous plant foods. To eat a high-meat diet today, you would be wise to also replicate this aspect of their diet or you risk a wide range of potential digestive problems. *Note: The safest way to enjoy your meat is to choose long, slow cooking methods (like stews, curries, and casseroles) and opt for rare or medium-rare when having a steak.*

5 WHAT ABOUT OFFAL?

If you truly want to eat like a hunter-gatherer, you will also have to broaden your palate past the juicy fillet and include marrow, heart, liver, kidney, brain, intestines, and so on. Our ancestors would almost certainly have used the entire animal carcass and been scavengers of food left over from other animal kills. There are many different nutrients to be found in these different body parts, but are you willing to try it?

6 WE DRIVE TO THE STORE TO HUNT!

The energy needs of hunter-gatherer man were very different. Enormous amounts of energy were expended in hunting and gathering food. It is estimated that today our energy needs are about half that of our far more active ancestors. There are two messages here—first, that our bodies are designed to be active and need activity to be healthy, and second, since most of us will never manage to replicate these extremely high levels of activity, our dietary needs are clearly different.

[TEXT CONTINUED]

The argument that we are genetically designed to eat a more animal-based diet is a valid one, and we can take some lessons from this. But we can also look at it from a different angle. As man's brain grew so did his capacity for thought and reasoning. We learned how to grow food and thus make it more available and sustainable. Human populations flourished and today the world population is around 6.5 billion people. We simply could not have grown to this number without grains and other carbohydrate-rich plants to use as food staples around the world, nor could we feed the world population today on a predominately animal-based diet. The fact is that most of the world survives on a carbohydrate-rich diet. Indeed many people around the world, out of choice or food availability, survive and thrive on a completely meat-free diet. One of our survival qualities has been that people can and do survive on a number of different diets depending on the availability of food around. There is not one diet to fit all—you can choose between a number of different healthy diets based on your personal circumstances, health, likes and dislikes, cost, and availability of food.

So if you think you would like to follow a diet more like that of our early ancestors, by all means do so, but this does not mean a low-carb diet. Cut back, or cut out, grain foods and instead seriously up your intake of vegetables and fruits. Choose a variety of lean cuts of different meats and include fish and seafood several times a week.

WHAT ABOUT SUGAR?

For years we've been told that sugar is bad and complex carbohydrates are good. Contrary to what "common sense" tells us, foods high in sugar do not have a high GI and those high in complex carbohydrates a low GI. In fact, very often the reverse is true. Sugar is just the name for short chain carbohydrates, while starch is a long-chain carbohydrate made up of individual sugars (glucose). Once broken down in the intestine and absorbed into the body, the individual glucose units are all the same whether they came from sugar or starch. The length of the carbohydrate chain doesn't tell us how fast it will hit the bloodstream. An apple is made up of sugars but has a low GI, whereas white bread is starch and has a high GI. The sugar content of these foods tells us nothing about their physiological effect. The key point is that refined and processed carbohydrates, whether they are starch, sugar, or a combination of both, are the problem.

Looking at the grams of sugar on the nutrition panel of a packaged food is not helpful because this figure does not distinguish between sugars that are naturally present in foods, such as in fruit, and sugar that is added to food. Table sugar is sugar refined from the sugar cane or sugar beet plant. It is really no different than white flour, which is the refined carbohydrate portion of the plant. Yet we don't have the same negative associations with flour as we do with sugar. From a glycemic impact point of view, flour is far worse. Table sugar is made up of two sugars — glucose and fructose. The latter does not have an immediate impact on blood glucose as it must first be metabolized by the liver. This is why many foods with added table sugar have low or intermediate

GIs. Flour, on the other hand, is made up of long chains of pure glucose and therefore most foods based on white flour have a high GI.

Nutritionally, eating a lot of table sugar is not a good idea. Table sugar is pure carbohydrate, providing energy and no other nutrients, hence you sometimes hear it referred to as "empty calories." If we are aiming to maximize our nutrient intake and control our energy intake, taking up "space" with table sugar is clearly not wise. However, sugar does have a place. It can make some very healthy foods more palatable. You and your children are far more likely to enjoy a bowl of oatmeal with a sprinkle of brown sugar than without it, and it's far healthier than white-bread toast. The bottom line is to look at the overall healthiness of a food rather than its sugar content. Foods with naturally present sugars are not bad for us and, in fact, are usually fabulous choices. A good idea is to use these foods as a sweetener rather than adding table sugar. For example, stir a fruit purée through natural yogurt for dessert instead of buying yogurts sweetened with table sugar or artificial sweeteners.

HONEY

Another natural alternative to using sugar is honey. Honey is enjoyed by native cultures all around the world and, since ancient times, honey has been used not just as a sweetener but also as a healing agent. Honey has many qualities that make it a better choice than table sugar — it has antimicrobial qualities (you can buy honey salves and dressings to help heal wounds), it contains antioxidants and other phytochemicals with health-promoting qualities, it contains small amounts of vitamins and minerals and, if you choose pure floral honeys rather than the supermarket blends, it has a low GI.

MAPLE SYRUP

Maple syrup is another reasonably good sugar alternative because it is a natural product. It is made by collecting the sap from the trunks of maple trees and boiling it for hours to reduce it to a syrup. The result is a delicious and low-GI sweetener. Don't confuse the real thing with maple-flavored syrup — this is less expensive but is also less nutritious, contains undesirable additives, and is not low GI.

Conclusions in the great carb debate

- We have eaten grain foods for several thousands of years without apparent ill effects and, in fact, our ability to survive on crops has sustained an increased world population. From an environmental point of view, we cannot all survive on a meat-dominated diet. The problems have only arisen with the increased consumption of heavily processed grain products which frequently have unhealthy additives.

- Whole grains and legumes provide us with key nutrients and fiber our bodies need.

- Whole grains and legumes are relatively cheap, readily available, and easy to store, making them invaluable as part of a modern healthy diet.

- The GI is an invaluable tool in helping us to make better choices about carbohydrate-rich foods.

- Hunter-gatherer man did not eat grains to any great extent but did have far greater quantities of vegetables and fruits than we do today. These ancestors also ate parts of the animal we may no longer find appetizing, and the nutrient profile of today's domesticated animals makes it hard, if not impossible, to truly replicate a hunter-gatherer diet. You can choose not to eat or at least reduce grain foods, but you must seriously up your intake of other plant foods instead.

So, after a thorough study of the evidence, limiting carbohydrates in your diet is not a path to a healthy lifelong diet. Focus on the quality and key nutritional aspects of the whole food instead.

World's Healthiest Carbohydrates ☆ ☆ ☆ ☆ ☆

The 5-star carbs give you sustained energy, brain power, concentration, intestinal health, and a good night's sleep. Each food was assigned a rating based on its nutritional profile. The criteria for the rating process were based on the food's ability to fuel the body for optimal performance. Consideration was given to GI, key nutrients, fiber content, antioxidants/phytochemicals, and numerous processing factors.

BARLEY

Barley is an ancient grain, one of the first to have been cultivated by man. It has been used as both a staple food and for medicinal purposes since biblical times. Unfortunately, today it has lost popularity as more readily available and processed grains are now the norm and the knowledge of how to prepare grains from their basic form has been lost.

Barley, like oats, is rich in soluble fiber and so can be effective in lowering blood cholesterol levels and contributes to good digestive health. Barley is a good source of many nutrients including the B-group vitamins, especially thiamin and niacin, iron, manganese, phosphorus, and potassium. It is available in several forms, most commonly as pearled barley, in which the bran and outer husk of the grain are removed. Unfortunately, this removes some of the fiber and results in the loss of nutrients. However, it is more palatable in this form and remains highly nutritious. Pot barley (sometimes called Scotch barley) is less refined and contains more of this bran layer. Most nutritious of all is hulled barley, where only the outer inedible husk is removed. Pearl barley is widely available but you may have

to look for pot or hulled barley in your local health food store. The good news is that all these forms of barley have a low GI and breads made with the cracked grains or intact kernels are also low GI. As with other grains, higher levels of processing increases the GI.

BEANS AND LENTILS (LEGUMES)

Beans and lentils truly are 5-star foods: They provide low-GI carbohydrates, are a plant source of protein and iron, are rich in soluble fiber, and they even provide a whole host of antioxidants and newly discovered phytochemicals being researched for their ability to protect us from a range of chronic diseases.

In the West they are often thought of as simply vegetarian fare, and indeed they are invaluable as a protein source in a meat-free diet, but legumes are excellent replacements for the more common high-GI carbs in a carnivorous diet.

The biggest hurdle for most people confronted with legumes is what to do with them. They are most often purchased as dried or ready to use in cans. The latter is more convenient as, with the exception of lentils and split peas, legumes require soaking before they are cooked. Cooking them yourself from their dried form may be more time consuming but is worthwhile as the beans retain more bite and extra flavor. However, for most purposes, the canned varieties are just as good. Instead of a bowl of fluffy white rice, which provides a small amount of readily absorbed carbohydrates, opt for a lentil dahl. Or make a chickpea mash to serve with grilled meat in place of mashed potatoes. A bean salsa is delicious with fish instead of boiled potatoes or bread rolls.

Judy swears that adding a strip of the sea vegetable kombu (available from Asian or health food stores) can improve the digestibility of the beans and help to prevent flatulence. Sea salt should only be added to the water in the last 5 minutes of cooking (otherwise the skin of the bean will never soften). Once cooked, skim off any froth, as this can also cause flatulence and discard the kombu.

The table below is a guide to cooking legumes and what to do with some of the more well-known varieties (unless stated otherwise, all beans require overnight soaking).

COOKING SUGGESTIONS FOR LEGUMES

LEGUME	DESCRIPTION	COOKING TIME	COOKING SUGGESTION
Adzuki beans	A small, red, sweet-flavored bean. Available in cans.	50 minutes–1 hour	Substitute for meat in casseroles. Popular in Japan.
Black-eyed peas	Mild-flavored bean, white with a black spot on the end. Available in cans.	1–1½ hours	Delicious with fish.
Black beans	Also called turtle beans. Available in cans.	2 hours	Popular in South America and delicious with spicy Mexican flavors and cool salsas. Delicious in casseroles and soups.
Cannellini beans	White beans of a similar size to kidney beans. Available in cans.	1–1½ hours	Delicious mashed with garlic as a potato substitute. Also good in dips.
Chickpeas (garbanzo beans)	Round, firm-bodied white bean. Popular in Moroccan cooking. Available in cans.	1–1½ hours	Widely used to make hummus. Chickpea flour (besan flour) is excellent for making savory pancakes.
Green (Puy) lentils (no soaking required)	Puy lentils are native to France and, like champagne, the name is controlled. The lentil is small and green with a delicious, nutty taste and holds its shape well.	20 minutes	Delicious in salads, or as a base for fish and lamb dishes.
Kidney beans	A stronger-tasting red bean. Available in cans.	1–1½ hours	Used in Mexican cooking. Well known in *chili con carne*.
Red lentils (no soaking required)	Small orange/red lentils. The archetypal vegetarian food.	15 minutes	Commonly used to make lentil soup. Delicious in lentil patties and dahl.
Lima beans	Also known as butter beans. A large white bean.	1–1½ hours	Serve in soups and winter casseroles.

BREADS

PUMPERNICKEL

Pumpernickel bread is a delicious, heavy, dark bread made from whole-grain rye flour and meal. It is low GI, filling, and comes in thin slices that are hard to overeat. It's available from most supermarkets, delis, and health food stores.

STONEGROUND

The name comes from the way in which the flour is ground — between pairs of stones rather than the more modern method using steel rollers. This produces a coarser flour with larger fiber particles giving the bread a lower GI. Using the whole grain also ensures that all the nutrients found in the grain make their way into the bread.

WHOLE-GRAIN AND RYE SOURDOUGH

The acidic sourdough starter, made by fermenting flour and water over a period of time to use in place of yeast, helps to reduce the GI of this dense and delicious bread. Even white sourdough has a low GI, but only whole-grain and rye sourdough varieties rate as 5-star foods because not only are they low GI but they're packed with fiber and micronutrients not found in plain white sourdough. Sourdough's popularity is increasing and you can now find many exceptional loaves in delis, health food stores, and produce markets all over the country.

WHOLE-GRAIN BREAD

Whole-grain bread (where there are lots of visible grain kernels) is both low GI and packed with fiber and micronutrients. Whole wheat is not the same thing — the fiber is so ground down as to make no real difference to the GI. Make sure you can make the distinction between the two when you are buying bread from the supermarket. Also note that multigrain is really just white flour mixed with a few grains and you cannot be sure of the GI unless it has been tested. Look for the low-GI symbol or buy one that's obviously heavy on grains.

BUCKWHEAT

Buckwheat is described as a grain but is in fact a seed related to sorrel and rhubarb. It has been a staple food for hundreds of years in Asia and Eastern Europe and is a worthy addition to your diet for several reasons. Unlike most whole grains, buckwheat is a rich source of all eight essential amino acids. This makes it a particularly good choice for vegetarians. It's also good for those with wheat or gluten intolerances because it is gluten-free and not related to wheat. It is high in fiber, promoting good digestive health, and has a low GI. It also tends to lower the GI of bread when added to a flour mix. That may be due, at least in part, to its soluble fiber content which may have further benefits in lowering blood cholesterol levels. Indeed, one Chinese study has shown that consumption of buckwheat was associated with a healthier blood cholesterol profile. Buckwheat is a good source of magnesium, important for healthy blood vessels, and may help to reduce blood pressure. It also contains a range of flavonoid antioxidants that may add to the grain's potential to protect the body from cardiovascular disease.

Buckwheat can be bought whole and cooked like rice or it can be roasted (roasted buckwheat is called kasha). You can also buy it as Japanese *soba* noodles or as flour, which is gray/brown in color. Buckwheat can also be used in a variety of baked goods, including pancakes, breads, and muffins. People suffering from celiac disease should avoid buckwheat noodles and pancake mix as they are usually blended with wheat flour. To cook whole buckwheat as an alternative to rice or potatoes, add 3 cups water to 1 cup buckwheat, bring to a boil before reducing the heat to a simmer, and cook for 30 minutes or until tender.

BULGUR

Bulgur is popular in Middle Eastern cuisine and is made from whole wheat. The whole kernels are steamed and dried before being cracked into pieces. As a result, it is sometimes known as cracked wheat. Because it is minimally processed, bulgur has a low GI, making it an excellent replacement for the more common high-GI carbohydrates in Western cuisine such as white rice and potatoes. Bulgur is a highly nutritious grain providing protein, niacin, thiamin, folate, and several minerals including iron, zinc, and calcium, and as a whole wheat product is high in the insoluble fiber important for good digestive health. As with other high-fiber grains, bulgur contains lignans, which are phytestrogens that have come under scientific interest for their involvement in protecting against certain cancers and possibly heart disease.

HOW TO PREPARE BULGUR

One great quality of bulgur is that it needs very little cooking. Place 1 cup of bulgur in a dish, cover with 2 cups of boiling water or stock and leave to soak for about 30 minutes, or until all the liquid is absorbed. If necessary, you can drain off any excess liquid.

You can buy bulgur in three different granulations — coarse, medium, and fine. You can find it in your local supermarket, sometimes in the ethnic food section or next to the rice, or in health food stores.

CORN (WHOLE)

Thank goodness for corn — often the only vegetable our children will eat! Nothing beats a sweet, succulent ear of corn, and when you use fresh corn that's sweet and juicy, there's really no need to slather it with butter. Corn was first discovered in Mexico where ears of corn were found in caves dating back as far as 5000 B.C. and corn remains a staple food throughout Mexico and Central America. Although thought of as a vegetable, corn is in fact a cereal and is rich in carbohydrates. We consider it to be a 5-star food first because it is low GI, providing a slow release of energy and helping to keep you full between meals. (Mexican corn tortillas are also low GI.) Second, when eaten on the cob it is easy to determine a portion size: One cob equals one serving. This makes it hard to overeat and a great alternative to potatoes in a meal. Finally, corn is a good source of many nutrients: fiber, vitamin C, phosphorus, manganese, and several B-group vitamins including thiamin and folate. The yellow color of corn comes from the carotenoid beta-cryptoxanthin. This antioxidant has been associated with a reduced risk of lung cancer (Mannisto et al, 2004) and rheumatoid arthritis (Cerhan et al, 2003).

When buying corn, check under the husks and avoid cobs with gaps and missing rows. The kernels should be plump, not withered, and husks should be fresh, pliable, and green. Corn is best during spring and summer — ready for barbecue season. Another advantage is how easy it is to cook; simply remove the husks and all remaining thin fibers and place it in a steamer to cook for 4 minutes until the corn is tender. This helps to preserve the water-soluble nutrients. Rather than smothering the cooked cobs in butter, try drizzling over a little olive or avocado oil. The fat does more than add flavor, it also increases the absorption of many nutrients including the carotenoids. Corn also cans well and is a convenient means of always having some on hand for use in sandwiches and salads, thrown into a Bolognese sauce or burger mix, or made into a quick salsa.

FREEKEH

Freekeh (pronounced free-ka), also known as farik, is an ancient Eastern Mediterranean grain. The story goes that in 2300 B.C., a nation in the Eastern Mediterranean picked the heads of their wheat harvest while it was still young and green because they needed to store food to see them through an expected siege on their walled city. During the conquest, the store of green wheat caught fire and the outer grains were burned. In an attempt to salvage their food store, they rubbed the heads of the wheat which exposed delicious toasted green grains.

HOW TO PREPARE FREEKEH

ABSORBPTION METHOD

1 cup Greenwheat freekeh

5 cups cold water

Bring to the boil in a large saucepan, simmer 20–25 minutes (cracked grain) or 45 minutes (whole grain).

MICROWAVE METHOD

1 cup Greenwheat freekeh

2 cups boiling water

Place in a deep microwave bowl, cover, and cook on high for 10 minutes (cracked grain and whole grain). Stand for 5 minutes.

Note: 1 cup dry freekeh yields 3 cups cooked freekeh.

They called the new style of grain "freekeh," meaning "the rubbed one" in their ancient Aramaic language.

Eastern Mediterranean people have eaten freekeh ever since and recently an Australian company developed a unique technology for producing this highly nutritious grain for mass consumption. However, it can be hard to find in the U.S. Look for freekeh in some health food stores or in Mediterranean specialty shops.

Nutritionally, freekeh is far superior to many other grains and the more common carbohydrate-rich foods we eat. Freekeh has up to four times the fiber of brown rice, provides more protein than mature wheat and most other grains — its protein content is similar to pasta made from durum wheat — and is rich in iron, zinc, potassium, and calcium. Freekeh is also high in resistance starch, which cannot be digested and absorbed in the small intestine and therefore reaches the colon where it acts like dietary fiber and contributes to bowel health. This also means the total carbohydrate load of the freekeh meal is reduced, particularly compared to a similar meal using rice or pasta. Not only that, but studies found both the cracked and whole-grain forms of freekeh to be low GI. All in all this makes freekeh hard to beat for those trying to manage their weight, prevent or manage diabetes, reduce the risk of heart disease, and promote good bowel health ... and that's just about all of us.

OATS AND NATURAL MUESLI

In Samuel Johnson's first dictionary of the English language, oats were defined as "eaten by people in Scotland, but fit only for horses in England." One Scotsman's retort to this was, "That's why England has such good horses, and Scotland has such fine men!"

The humble oat is hard to beat when it comes to a complete nutritional package. Not only do oats provide energy-sustaining, low-GI carbohydrates, but they are also relatively high in protein. In fact, about 12 percent of the energy in oats comes from protein, making them an especially valuable grain for vegetarians. The fat in oats is high for a grain, providing about 20 percent of the total energy, but this is almost all healthy unsaturated fat. The fat present also carries fat-soluble vitamin E, a key player in the team of disease-fighting antioxidants in the body. In fact, a half-cup of raw oats provides roughly 20 percent of the recommended daily intake (RDI) of vitamin E for women, and 15 percent than for

NATURAL MUESLI

Oats are the main ingredient in muesli. When you are buying a ready-made muesli from the supermarket or health food store, always check the packaging for added sugar. Sugar listed on the nutritional panel applies to both the sugar naturally present in the fruits and added sugar so always check the ingredients. Choose one with no added sugar or oil. Alternatively, make your own using your favorite ingredients or try the recipe on page 160.

men. Oats provide a whole host of other micronutrients including the B-group vitamins, potassium, calcium, magnesium, phosphorus, iron, zinc, manganese, and the antioxidant mineral selenium.

Along with barley, oats are among the best grain sources of soluble fiber and are renowned for their cholesterol-lowering abilities. Taken together, these attributes make oats a star performer in preventing cardiovascular disease.

Rolled oats are the most commonly available form in the U.S. The nutritious outer husk is relatively intact as the grain is lightly steamed and pressed into flat flakes. These are perfect for making your own granola or muesli, or for a quick oatmeal. Don't be tempted to buy instant oats — they may take less time to prepare but are less nutritious with added sugar and flavorings, have a higher GI, and won't keep you feeling full for as long. Besides, rolled oats will cook in a few minutes — how much quicker do we need breakfast to be?

Coarse oats or steel-cut oats are roughly cut groats (the whole grain). They undergo little processing and consequently are an excellent source of fiber and nutrients. Traditional oatmeal involves soaking the grain overnight and cooking it in water with a pinch of salt for up to 45 minutes. As not many people have so much time to spend first thing in the morning, you could save it for the weekend or invest in a slow cooker. Left to cook overnight, you wake to instant oatmeal for a fraction of the GI of quicker cooking methods. Rolled and steel-cut oats are readily available at supermarkets and health food stores.

Oats will remain fresh stored in an airtight container in a cool pantry for most of the year, but during the hotter summer months they are best stored in the fridge. Use within three months of purchase.

QUINOA

Quinoa (pronounced keen-wa) is a tiny South American grain that has been cultivated for more than 5000 years and was a staple food of the ancient Incas. It is sometimes referred to as a "supergrain" given its superior nutrient profile compared to other grains, although it is not really a grain but the seed of a leafy plant. Quinoa is relatively high in protein and, most importantly, the protein is of superior quality because it provides the amino acid lysine which is missing in most grains. This makes it an excellent inclusion in a vegetarian diet. Quinoa also has a low GI, and is a good source of iron, potassium, and B-group vitamins. It is becoming more widely available as

HOW TO PREPARE QUINOA

Quinoa is naturally coated in a bitter compound called saponin. The quinoa you purchase in stores has already had the saponin washed away, but you should give the grains a good rinse under the cold tap to remove any residue. Place the quinoa in a saucepan with one part grain to two parts water. Bring to a boil, reduce to a simmer, cover, and cook until the grains become translucent and you can see the spiral germ on each grain. This should take about 15 minutes. You can also toast the quinoa before cooking to give it a nuttier, roasted flavor. Simply heat a nonstick frying pan, and toast the grain for about 5 minutes. Cook as above.

it gains in popularity from health savvy consumers. You will find it in health food stores and the grains section of many supermarkets.

WHOLE-WHEAT PASTA

With four times the iron content and over double the zinc, whole-wheat pasta is more nutritionally valuable than white pasta. Both have a low GI compared to other traditionally popular carbohydrates, but with whole-wheat providing over three times the fiber content of white pasta, it's worth adjusting to the taste.

Whole-wheat pasta cooks in the same way as white but takes almost twice as long. It has a nuttier flavor so that many people, having made the switch for health reasons, refuse to go back to white pasta because they prefer the taste of whole-wheat.

Look for pastas (and breads) made from the ancient grains spelt or Kamut®. Both claim to be better tolerated by people who are sensitive to modern, hybrid wheats with high gluten content. Spelt and Kamut® are nutritionally superior, boasting far higher protein and micronutrient contents. They taste fantastic but the downside is they also cost more.

PROTEINS

WORLD'S HEALTHIEST PROTEINS

☆ ☆ ☆ ☆ ☆

Chicken and Turkey, skin removed

Eggs, free range or organic

Fish, especially oily

Game Meats (for example, venison)

Lean Pork

Lean Red Meat

Liver

Low-Fat Milk and Natural Yogurt

Seafood (except for prawns, squid, and fish roe)

Protein is found throughout the body — in the hair, skin, nails, teeth, bone, every internal organ, and, in fact, virtually every cell. Proteins are also used as chemical messengers, enzymes, and nutrient carriers in the blood. It's easy to see why protein is so important in our diet. The question is, how much is optimal for our health and does it matter where we get it from?

The question of how much is not easy to answer. We certainly know how much we roughly need on a daily basis to balance how much we lose: less than 1 gram of protein for about every 2 pounds of body weight. Since the body doesn't have spare stores of protein, like it does for carbohydrates and fat, failing to meet your requirement will mean your body has to pull protein from other parts of the body — usually muscle.

The effects of not getting enough protein are apparent in many parts of the developing world. Protein malnutrition, called kwashiorkor, results in growth failure in children, a loss of muscle mass, decreased immunity, a weakening of the heart and respiratory system and, ultimately, death. In the developed world where a variety of foods are readily available, meeting the physiological requirement for protein is easy. Defining the upper limit for intake is far more difficult.

High-protein diets first appeared in the 1960s but then lost popularity in the wake of the low-fat diet era that followed. The failure of the latter to curb our rising tide of overweight people, obesity, and chronic disease has led to a striking comeback for high-protein diets. The scientific community were at first slow to respond, and most refuted the claims made. However, in the last few years, there has been renewed interest and evidence is emerging to give us a better picture of protein's place in our diet.

There is now convincing evidence to show that a higher amount of protein in the diet can help you to lose weight, improve body composition, help prevent regaining weight and be beneficial for your heart (Krieger et al, 2006; Halton and Hu, 2004). *What this does not mean is that carbs are bad and proteins, whatever the source, are good.* The key aspect seems to be more protein, and the diet does not have to be low carbohydrate. Furthermore, there are real concerns over long-term effects on those following low-carb/high-protein diets (Trichopoulou, 2007; Lagiou et al, 2007) with at least two recent prospective studies, one from Greece and the other from Sweden, reporting increased mortality, particularly from cardiovascular disease.

Popular diet books tend to make nutrition all black and white with no shades of gray. They list good and bad foods with "easy" rules on how to follow the diet, but there is no evidence to support the safety or efficacy of these diets in the long term. High-protein diets are not all the same; some have high fat levels, some have high fat but low saturated fat and, they may be low carbohydrate while others have a more moderate amount of carbohydrates and so on. Results from studies done on these diet plans are never the same, and we can't dismiss the enormous amount of scientific evidence we have concerning fats, fiber, fruits, vegetables, whole grains, and so on. For optimum health, we need to pull all the evidence together to make sensible conclusions about the best diet.

The person who lives mostly on modern high-GI carbohydrates will tend to have large fluctuations in blood glucose (sugar) and a correspondingly high insulin demand on the body. High triglycerides (blood fat), low (good) HDL-cholesterol, high insulin, and glucose "spikes" after meals are all a recipe for disaster, increasing the risk of heart disease, type 2 diabetes and related conditions. This does not happen when you choose minimally processed low-GI carbohydrates and/or *some* carbohydrates are replaced with protein.

Protein can assist in weight control in a number of ways:

- Protein takes more energy (more calories) to digest and metabolize than carbohydrates or fat.

- Protein is very satiating and can help to prevent hunger pangs between meals.

More protein and fewer carbohydrates reduce the glycemic load and therefore the subsequent rise in blood glucose. This in turn reduces the amount of insulin required to deal with the incoming "meal." With less insulin there is less likely to be a dramatic drop in blood glucose levels that can stimulate hunger 1–2 hours after the meal. And since insulin is a storage hormone — its job is to stimulate the absorbsion of incoming fat, carbohydrates, and protein into cells in muscles, liver, and adipose tissue (fat stores) — less insulin around means less stimulus for fat storage and allows for greater fat burning.

But remember, this does not mean you need to cut carbs completely and neither can you ignore the type of fat you're eating. The best evidence supports replacing refined carbohydrates with protein that is low in saturated fat or with low-GI whole grains or a combination of the two.

Can too much protein be harmful?

Yes. The early explorers of the Americas quickly learned that if they ate only rabbits and few other foods, they got extremely sick and many died. They called this condition "rabbit starvation." Lean meat alone provided them with excessive protein and little carbohydrate or fat. We have a finite ability to metabolize protein, and overloading the system results in acid build-up in the blood and, ultimately, death.

To a lesser extreme, eating a lot of protein, particularly animal protein, leads to acidic urine which the kidneys neutralize with calcium. The increase in calcium in the urine is well documented among those following higher-protein diets. What is not known is whether this calcium comes from better absorption of calcium from the foods in this diet — and certainly there is some evidence that this occurs when the protein comes from animal foods but not from supplements — or whether the calcium is coming from bone. While the jury is still out on the reason, the risk is not worth taking given the debilitating and painful condition of osteoporosis. A point to note is that our ancestors, despite their high-protein diet, appeared to have had extremely strong skeletons. This protection was probably due to their consumption of large quantities of plant foods which buffer the acidity without drawing on calcium stores (Barzel and Massey, 1998). Of course, they were also far more active than we are today and exercise is crucial for healthy, strong bones. There are two lessons we can learn here. First, yes we can choose to eat a higher protein diet, but it must be accompanied by plentiful quantities of plant foods. Second, our bodies were built to be active and we absolutely must build exercise into our lives if we want the best health.

A CASE FOR EATING ANIMAL FOODS

We have only to look at our requirement for certain nutrients for pretty compelling evidence of our need for animal foods:

- **IRON** — daily requirement is 18 milligrams for women (19–50 years of age) and 8 milligrams for all men and women over the age of 50. It is difficult to meet these requirements with plant foods alone. The best sources of readily absorbable iron are liver, red meat, seafood, and other animal foods. By contrast, the iron found in plant foods is poorly absorbed, although helped somewhat by the presence of vitamin C, and the body has the ability to increase absorption when iron is needed. Iron is necessary for transporting oxygen around the body, in the production of energy to complete physical work, and in maintaining a healthy immune system. The symptoms of low iron intake therefore include fatigue, inability to exercise, an intolerance of the cold, and frequent colds, flu, and other infections.

- **ZINC** — daily requirement is 8 milligrams for women and 14 milligrams for men. While the outer husk of grains does contain some zinc, other plant sources are generally low in this mineral. Animal foods are our best source, with seafood and red meat being particularly zinc-rich. Zinc is essential for energy production, for maintaining a healthy immune system, for healthy sperm production in men, for normal growth and development in children, and for healthy teeth, bones, and skin. A lack of zinc can lead to skin problems, reproductive defects, immune deficiency, eye problems, and osteoporosis.

- **VITAMIN B12** — only found in animal foods. We are very efficient at recycling this vitamin and so it takes many years of a strict vegan diet to develop a deficiency. Nevertheless, the fact that a nutrient found only in animal foods is so essential to the functioning of the human body is indicative of the fact that we are meant to eat animal food in some form. Vitamin B12 is essential for the conversion of food into energy, in protein and fat metabolism, for a healthy nervous system, for good skin and hair, in the production of DNA, and for normal growth and development.

- **TAURINE** — an amino acid required for successful synthesis of proteins throughout the body. While we can make taurine from other amino acids, there is some evidence that our ability to do this is fairly limited. Taurine is only available in our diet from animal food sources, further adding to the argument that we need animal proteins.

- **VITAMIN A** — an important antioxidant and essential for healthy function of the eyes, yet this vitamin is not found in any plant food. It is true that certain carotenoids, including beta-carotene, found widely in plant foods, can be converted to vitamin A in the liver. However, our capacity to do so is limited.

The types of fat available to us from plant and animal sources are different. Only animal foods have the longer-chain fats essential for the normal functioning of all cells in the body. While we can make these longer-chain fats from the shorter plant fats, we are less efficient at doing so. This applies to the omega-3 fats we know to be important in brain development and function — those present in plants such as flaxseeds are shorter chains than those found in oily fish and do not have quite the same effect. (They are still beneficial and a good option for those who can't or won't eat fish and/or seafood.)

This is not to say that you cannot follow a vegetarian diet. You can indeed do so, provided you take great care in your food choices to provide all the nutrients you need. The stricter you are with the foods you avoid, the harder this becomes. If you choose to follow a vegan diet, you would do well to use animal-free supplements to ensure you meet all nutrient requirements. What this evidence does suggest is that, genetically, humans have evolved to rely on animal produce for key essential nutrients. If you choose to be vegetarian or vegan, do so for personal, moral, or religious reasons, but not with the belief that it will necessarily be healthier. Equally, it is clearly important for meat eaters to be discerning about the protein foods they eat regularly and they must also be sure to include enough plant foods to balance their diets.

Type of protein

The building blocks of protein are the amino acids, of which around 20 are important in the human metabolism. Every protein in the body is made from particular combinations of the amino acids. Some of these we can synthesize from other amino acids, while some must be obtained from our diet. The latter are called the essential amino acids. The protein in our food contains various quantities of amino acids. Animal foods, including dairy foods, contain all of the essential amino acids and are known as complete proteins. Plant foods, in contrast, almost always lack or are low in one or more of the essential amino acids. This is not a problem provided a variety of different plant foods are consumed throughout the day. For example, grains are low in the amino acid lysine, but if you eat your bread with hummus or lentil spread you will obtain your lysine from this source. These are sometimes called "complementary proteins." The exception is soy protein. This does contain all of the essential amino acids and, for this reason, is often used in protein powders and is an alternative infant formula for babies intolerant to cows' milk. If you are vegetarian, soy beans and soy products such as tofu and tempeh are smart additions to your diet.

We must also pay attention to the other nutrients that come along with the protein in foods. Many animal-sourced, protein-rich foods are also fat-rich foods, and much of this fat is saturated.

Only a few of the currently popular high-protein diets recognize this and make specific recommendations about the type of fat. The vast majority of diets have pushed the low-carbohydrate ideal without consideration as to the quality of the foods that remain. This is exactly the same mistake as was made early on with the low-fat era of dietary recommendations. We must stop these ridiculous, one-eyed diets that blame one macronutrient for all our ailments. When choosing foods we should be more concerned with the quality and nutritional value of the food rather than obsessing over the macronutrient content. The bottom line is that we need quality carbohydrates, quality fats, and quality proteins to look, feel, and perform at our best.

World's Healthiest Proteins ☆ ☆ ☆ ☆ ☆

CHICKEN AND TURKEY

Chicken has become such a popular meat that chicken producers have, of course, searched for ways to produce greater quantities of meat for a cheaper price. There have been numerous scare stories in the media. In particular, there is a widespread belief that chickens are fed hormones to promote rapid growth and that this is causing horrendous health effects in both children and adults. However, according to USDA regulations, the use of hormones in chicken has been banned since the 1952. *Regardless of which type of chicken you choose to purchase, be assured that it does not contain growth-promoting hormones.* Nevertheless, while it could be argued that from a nutritional standpoint there are few differences between birds raised free range or in an intensive farming practice, undeniably the former tastes infinitely better and, from a humane standpoint, the birds have lived a happier life. So just what is the difference between conventional, free range, and organic?

CONVENTIONAL, COMMERCIALLY PRODUCED CHICKEN

Birds are raised in large sheds (they are not kept in cages) and do not have access to outdoor areas. The area or range per bird is considerably smaller than free range or organic methods.

While no hormones are given to the birds, antibiotics are often used although under strict industry codes. When antibiotics are used, strict USDA and FDA regulations require that the chickens are weaned from the antibiotics before they are processed so there are no antibiotics or antibiotic residues in the chicken you buy from the market. However, even some conventional chicken farms are looking for alternatives to antibiotics because of consumer concern. Concerns have been voiced over whether the use of antibiotics in chicken farming increases the numbers of antibiotic-resistant strains of bacteria, which may threaten human health. However, provided you prepare and cook chicken products correctly, all bacteria, resistant or otherwise, are killed making any cross-contamination extremely unlikely. In addition, the antibiotics used are not the same as those used in humans, although these are permitted when there is no alternative for treating a specific problem.

Finally, the feed used varies. For commercially reared birds, feed is predominantly grain-based, and pesticides, insecticides, and artificial fertilizers are likely to have been used, and it may also contain genetically modified crops.

FREE-RANGE CHICKEN

The major difference between free-range chickens and conventionally raised chickens is in their living conditions. Birds are allowed access to an outdoor run during the day and the area or range per bird is considerably larger than for conventional, commercially reared birds. The other major difference is that, in buying free-range chickens, you can be assured that antibiotics have not been used at any stage in the birds' life. Antibiotics can be given to treat disease, but the meat from these birds can no longer be sold as free range. The feeding practices are similar to conventional, commercially reared birds. The USDA is the certifying body for free-range chicken meat and all certified meat must comply with their standards.

ORGANIC CHICKEN

Organic chicken comes from birds with similar living conditions to free range; that is, they have access to an outdoor run during daylight hours and have far more space than conventional, commercially reared birds. The key differences here are that the feed used must be 95 percent organically certified. This means no genetically modified crops and no pesticide and insecticide use. Second, the birds can neither be treated with antibiotics and nor are they routinely vaccinated. Producers must comply with the USDA organic certification regulations and bear a certification label from an approved organization.

In deciding which type of chicken meat you buy, price will undoubtedly be a factor; conventional chickens are the cheapest and organic produce costs up to three times as much. The reason is quite simply that the organic farming method costs more — more space per bird and more expensive feed. We wholeheartedly support the organic philosophy and believe that this is the best option when possible, taking all factors including animal welfare into account not to mention taste. From a nutritional point of view, there may be small differences. Allowing birds to roam outside and feed on grass as nature intended can increase the omega-3 and vitamin-E content of the meat and eggs. Nevertheless, put the additional benefits of organic produce versus perceived dangers of conventional into perspective. There is little point in spending the extra on organic chicken for your family if you then also load the shopping cart with packages of cookies and bottles of soda, and stop on the way home for a fast-food burger!

EGGS

Eggs were once in, then they were out, and now no one really knows where they stand. Are eggs healthy or not? Well, the confusion has come about because of the many sides to the humble egg. On one hand, the egg comes pretty close to being the perfect food, providing many of our required nutrients. The egg white is almost entirely protein and contains all of the essential amino acids we need, while the yolk contains numerous vitamins and minerals (so please don't throw it away!). On the other hand, they are high in cholesterol and the yolk is a

WHAT'S IN AN EGG?

1 medium-sized egg (48 grams) provides:

70 calories

5.3 grams fat, of which 1.4 grams is saturated fat

206 milligrams cholesterol

0.1 gram carbohydrate

6.2 grams protein

considerable source of fat, providing 65 percent of the total energy of the whole egg.

EGG DEFINITIONS

CAGE EGGS
These eggs account for most eggs sold in the U.S. They come from hens kept in battery-style cages with little room or freedom for movement.

VEGETARIAN-FED EGGS
Most consumers see "vegetarian" and assume that therefore this is a healthier egg. In fact, in order for eggs to be vegetarian, the hens must be on a completely animal-product-free diet and this means they cannot be allowed to roam free range where they naturally forage for insects and worms outdoors. These eggs are therefore usually from cage-kept hens that are simply fed a vegetarian diet.

BARN-LAID EGGS
These are from hens that are housed in a large shed rather than cages. They have enough room to walk around and flap their wings, but do not have the same space as free-range birds.

OMEGA-3 EGGS
These are from hens fed a diet high in omega-3 fats and vitamin E to boost the content of these essential nutrients in the eggs. These may be either free-range or cage-kept hens—read the label to be sure. Those labeled "naturally richer in omega-3s" are usually from hens allowed to roam free range and consume a more natural diet including grass.

FREE-RANGE EGGS
These are from hens with access to an outdoor run during daylight hours. The hens therefore have more space than cage-kept hens. Behind organic eggs, free-range eggs enriched with omega-3s are the next best choice.

ORGANIC EGGS
These are eggs from hens fed certified-organic feed grown without the use of pesticides, insecticides, and artificial fertilizers. The hens cannot be fed antibiotics and conditions must comply with strict humane-practice codes. These eggs tend to be naturally richer in many nutrients including omega-3 fats and vitamin E due to the high quality of feed used. They will, however, be more expensive as a result.

When it was first realized that blood cholesterol levels were related to heart disease, it seemed a logical jump to assume that cholesterol in foods would have a major impact on blood cholesterol levels. This led to the advice to eat less cholesterol, and eggs hit the "bad" foods list. Add to this the obsession with eating low-fat foods, and eggs certainly lost favor. However, scientific research later showed that the major dietary influence on blood cholesterol is saturated fat and that dietary cholesterol has far less impact. The reason for this is that cholesterol in the blood comes from both diet and cholesterol produced in the liver — if you eat less cholesterol your liver will produce more and vice versa. Saturated fat, on the other hand, affects how much cholesterol the liver produces. Therefore, current dietary advice to maintain healthy cholesterol levels focuses on reducing saturated fat and replacing it with healthier unsaturated fats.

Eggs contain around 5 grams of fat each, but less than half of this comes from saturated fat. The type of egg you buy further influences the type of fats present. Free-range eggs may have a healthier fat profile than cage eggs. One study compared the nutrient profile of eggs from a U.S. supermarket (from battery hens fed a commercial feed) with those from a Greek village (free-range hens fed a traditional grain diet) and they found a phenomenal difference in the type of fats present. The Greek eggs contained less saturated fat and far more of the healthy fats, especially the omega-3 fats (Simopoulos and Salem, 1989). These are known to reduce your risk of heart attack, are important in maintaining healthy blood, and are essential for brain development and function. The feed given to the hens is clearly a crucial factor here and certainly you can now purchase cage eggs high in omega-3s. However, since we also know that exercise affects the fat levels in meat, this may also make a difference to the fats found in eggs; free-range hens are clearly more active than caged hens. This subject is hotly debated, with egg producers arguing that an egg is an egg. We say free-range hens must be happier and this is reason enough to buy their eggs. If we also get better nutrition, so much the better.

So, not only are eggs not "bad" but they can make a significant healthy contribution to your diet. If you already have high blood cholesterol it is probably best to limit yourself to around 4 per week but, otherwise, if you like to have eggs for breakfast then go ahead and enjoy. But be careful with the added extras — butter in scrambled eggs or cheese in an omelet can add a lot of the wrong kind of fat. Otherwise, go for poached or boiled eggs and add your choice of wilted spinach, grilled tomatoes, mushrooms, and whole-grain or sourdough bread. Delicious!

FISH

All fish is rated 5 stars because it is low in saturated fats and a good source of many nutrients including niacin and other B-group vitamins required for energy metabolism. Fish also provides iodine, an essential component of thyroid hormones; iron, for healthy red blood cells and oxygen transport; zinc, essential for many metabolic processes and a strong immune system; and small quantities of folate, essential in the production of DNA and new cells in the body.

Oily fish gets a special mention because these are the best sources of the omega-3 fats we now know to be more than just good for us, but essential for looking, feeling, and performing our best. Oily fish include salmon, trout, mackerel, sardines, tuna, and herring. Omega-3 fats help to prevent blood clots and thus reduce your risk of heart attack and stroke. They also have an anti-inflammatory effect and research has shown benefit to those with rheumatoid arthritis. Upping your intake of omega-3s from fish may also help in other inflammatory-related or auto-immune conditions including asthma, pulmonary disease, multiple sclerosis, psoriasis, and inflammatory bowel disease. For more information on omega-3 fats see page 78.

MERCURY IN FISH

One concern with increasing fish consumption is the mercury content. Increasing levels of mercury in our waters has occurred through industrial pollution and this mercury then builds up in the flesh of certain fish. All fish contain some traces of mercury, but it is the larger fish at the top of the food chain, or those with a longer life span, that accumulate higher levels. The greatest risk is to unborn children, infants, and young children. In babies, high exposure to mercury seems to, albeit subtly, affect attention, memory, and learning. For this reason, women planning a pregnancy and those who are pregnant should take care with which fish they consume on a regular basis. (Very little mercury is transferred in breast milk.) In adults it takes a lot more mercury to cause any symptoms — tingling in the lips, fingers, and toes is usually the first sign — but this is extremely unlikely to occur as a result of eating fish within health guidelines. The EPA regularly updates its recommendations and advisories on which fish and shellfish are safe and are recommended to eat as part of a healthy diet.

DID YOU KNOW?

3 ounces of cooked octopus has more than double the iron content of 3 ounces of cooked lean beef, but has 30 percent fewer calories and only a trace of saturated fat (compared to approximately 3 grams in lean beef) while both provide similar amounts of protein.

A dozen oysters is not only an elegant (and hopefully romantic) entrée, but provides almost 10 times the daily recommended intake for zinc, half that for iron and niacin, about a third for magnesium, and almost all the phosphorus an adult needs. All this for only 130 calories and 4 grams of fat.

A dozen mussels provide your total daily requirement for iron, a third that for zinc, more than a third of your magnesium, and a tenth of your vitamin-A needs, while providing only 130 calories, almost no saturated fat, and less than 3 grams total fat.

Half a medium-sized lobster provides only 150 calories, just over 1 gram of fat, and almost no saturated fat while supplying 32 grams of protein. Compare this to a medium-sized chicken breast (skin removed) with 260 calories, 11 grams of fat, of which 3 grams is saturated fat, and only a few more grams of protein. The lobster also provides seven times the iron and more than double the zinc of the chicken breast.

GAME MEATS

Game meats include emu, ostrich, venison, hare, rabbit, goat, buffalo (bison), quail, pigeon, partridge, grouse, pheasant, and guinea fowl. You have probably never tasted or even seen some of these meats and not all are readily available in the U.S. However, many are becoming more common on menus at fine restaurants. You should also be able to find several of the other game meats in many grocery stores and specialty butcher shops, and it is worth experimenting with these new tastes and flavors in your journey to better health.

So, why are game meats so fabulous? These are the closest meats we can find today to match those eaten by our hunter-gatherer ancestors. Although most are now farmed to some degree, this is far less intensive than the more popular domesticated animals and many continue to be "hunted" in the wild. This means antibiotics and hormones are not used, they eat their native diet, and they exercise far more than their domesticated relatives. As a result, game meat is generally incredibly lean, almost without exception low in saturated fat, a good source of omega-3 fats, high in protein, and comes with none of the concerns surrounding the intensive rearing of farm animals. The downside is that, because it's harder to find, less popular, and less intensively reared, game meats can also be more expensive (although not necessarily, so shop around).

Whichever meat you choose, we always advocate choosing quality over quantity. Use the money you save from cutting down on commercial packaged foods to spend on fresh quality foods such as this. So, don't compare the price of an elk fillet to a bag of processed meat sausages — in terms of "bang for your buck" the elk wins hands down and your body will thank you for it.

Note: Meats with low fat content can lose moisture and toughen quickly if exposed to high, dry cooking. The meat should be marinated before roasting or cooked in wet dishes.

COMPARING MEATS

PER 3.5 OZ. COOKED MEAT	ENERGY IN CALORIES	PROTEIN (grams)	FAT (grams)	SATURATED FAT (grams)	IRON (milligrams)	ZINC (milligrams)
venison	158	32.9	2.8	1.2	4.8	3.3
goat*	143	27.1	3.0	0.9	3.7	5.3
rabbit	170	29.3	5.7	2.2	1.3	2.1
beef rump	183	28.5	7.6	3.4	3.4	4.5
pork tenderloin	156	30.9	3.5	1.4	1.5	2.5
lamb (trimmed)	179	30.5	6.2	2.7	5.4	4.8
veal	142	31.6	1.6	0.5	1.8	3.7
quail	197	27.7	9.6	2.5	1.8	1.3
emu	123	25.7	2.2	0.7	2.9	1.0
ostrich*	111	32.2	1.2	1.0	4.9	4.9
chicken breast (no skin)	157	28.1	5.0	2.3	0.8	1.4
turkey breast (no skin)	155	29.4	4.0	0.9	0.6	1.9
duck (no skin)	182	24.3	9.5	2.8	2.6	2.9
liver, lamb	232	30.6	10.7	3.1	8.1	5.5
liver, chicken	159	25.7	5.5	1.8	7.3	4.0

Note: Analyzed using Foodworks Professional (Xyris software 2005) using Australian and New Zealand data.
*Figures from USDA database only.

All of these meats make a valuable contribution to a healthy diet. They are all relatively low in saturated fat, some extremely so, they provide similar amounts of good quality complete protein, and all are a source of the essential minerals iron and zinc. That said, some meats stand out as truly exceptional choices. Venison, goat, emu, and ostrich are very low fat and low saturated fat, but they have exceptionally good levels of iron and zinc, for relatively few calories. Ostrich is growing in popularity in both the U.S. and Europe as consumers become aware of its phenomenally healthy profile. If you get the chance to try it, do take the opportunity.

Unfortunately, many of us are not big fans of liver, while liver products such as pâté tend to have added undesirable fats such as butter and cream. A word of warning for pregnant

[TEXT CONTINUED]

women who need an iron boost: Liver contains a massive amount of vitamin A — almost 4500 times the recommended daily adult intake in lamb liver and almost 900 times in chicken liver! Such enormous amounts can be damaging to the developing fetus and for this reason all pregnant women should avoid liver and liver products. For everyone else, if you like it, an occasional liver meal will give you an incredible nutrient boost.

Of the more common, widely available meats, you can see that all of the lean cuts listed make pretty good choices. Sirloin steak or fillet and trimmed lamb cuts are the best for iron and zinc but beware that if you choose fattier cuts the saturated fat content can jump four-fold. Veal is very low in saturated fat and an excellent source of zinc. Chicken and, particularly, turkey breast are great protein sources with very little saturated fat, but these have far lower levels of iron and zinc. Duck tends to be much fattier, but if you remove the skin the saturated fat content is on a par with lean cuts of red meat and you get more iron and zinc than the other poultry options.

LEAN PORK

Apparently pork is the most widely eaten meat in the world, although in the West beef tends to be more popular. There are, of course, religious restrictions for some that will negate its place on our list. Note that we don't include pork products such as ham and bacon in the 5-star category, but fresh, lean pork cuts such as tenderloin are listed. This ensures that you get top-quality protein with very little total or saturated fat. Pork is also incredibly rich in the B vitamin thiamin, necessary to convert our food into energy for use by the body, and essential for normal growth and development and to maintain healthy functioning of the heart, the nervous system, and the digestive system.

LEAN RED MEAT

While obvious nutrient deficiencies are relatively uncommon in the developed world, one we often see is iron deficiency. This is in part due to our body's relatively high requirements for iron and the fact that so many of us simply don't eat enough iron-rich foods. Children and both pre-menopausal and pregnant women are particularly at risk given their higher requirements for the mineral. People also have increased requirements if they regularly give blood, have any sort of intestinal bleed (for example, an ulcer), or are recovering from an accident in which they lost a substantial amount of blood. Zinc is another mineral we have relatively high requirements for but is often low in diets, particularly when no meat is eaten.

Red meats, as we can see in the Comparing Meats table on page 63, are without doubt the best sources of both of these minerals and this is the major reason why we rate them in the 5-star category. If you choose lean cuts and trim away any visible fat, you get all the protein, iron, and zinc with only small amounts of saturated fat. It is well worth finding a good butcher in your area who stocks grass-fed (may be listed as pasture-fed) meat rather than grain-fed. The latter are fattened up on grain meal to encourage marbling of the meat — that is, fatty streaks throughout the meat which are impossible to remove. Chefs may well choose this type of meat as the fat helps to keep the meat moist and undoubtedly adds flavor, but if you want to keep your saturated fat intake down, go for the grass-fed, lean option. You just have to be more careful with cooking methods and you will find this type of meat to be delicious and incredibly nutritious.

LIVER

Liver is not to everyone's taste, including ours we must confess! However, there is no denying that liver is packed with essential nutrients including all the amino acids we need. In particular, liver is the best animal source of iron, containing 7–8 milligrams per 100 grams of meat, roughly double that of most red meats. It is also rich in zinc, necessary for a strong immune system and often lacking in modern diets, and a very good source of vitamin C, riboflavin, niacin, vitamin B6, pantothenic acid, folate, vitamin B12, phosphorus, copper, and selenium. Liver is extremely rich in vitamin A. This is good for most of us as it is necessary for good vision, among other things. However, since high levels of vitamin A can cause deformities during fetal development, pregnant women should avoid liver and liver products, including pâté. It can be quite fatty depending on the source (lamb's liver has more than double the fat of chicken liver), and be careful with liver products such as pâté, which have significant added fat, much of it saturated. It is also high in cholesterol. This is not a problem for most people because their saturated fat intake is far more likely to affect their blood cholesterol levels than how much dietary cholesterol they eat, but people with high cholesterol should limit their intake of pâté. Despite these flaws, we feel liver has to be a 5-star food given the rich nutrient mix it has to offer. Furthermore, if you believe in trying to follow a diet as close to our ancestors as possible, it's fairly certain liver would have been a prized food.

LOW-FAT MILK AND NATURAL YOGURT

Milk is considered such an important food in Western countries that, along with the various dairy products made from it, it merits a food group all to itself. Yet the vast majority of the rest of the world does not drink milk beyond infant-hood. This paradox has led to furious debates on the healthfulness of milk with fervent believers on both sides.

On a positive note, milk packs a whole lot of nutrition into one easy-to-consume and inexpensive package. The nutrients present include calcium, vitamin D, vitamin A, vitamin B12, niacin, riboflavin, potassium, phosphorus, good-quality protein providing all the essential amino acids we need, and low-GI carbohydrates. The fat in whole milk is high in saturated fats, but that's easy to avoid by choosing a low-fat milk from the vast range available.

Of all the health claims about milk, the one that probably comes to mind is that drinking milk is good for your bones. The risk of osteoporosis is increased in those with a low calcium intake, and it's hard to beat dairy products for easily absorbable calcium. Add to this the fact that vitamin D and phosphorus are also crucial for maintaining strong bones and milk does indeed look pretty good. You can, of course, get your calcium elsewhere, and in parts of Asia where they consume no dairy products and have far smaller daily intakes of calcium, they also have less osteoporosis. However, there are many other differences that may account for this including higher activity levels, genetic factors, and daily exposure to sunlight (needed to stimulate vitamin D production in the skin). Nevertheless, if you don't like, can't, or don't want to consume dairy products, you can obtain your calcium from dark green leafy vegetables, dried beans, fish (where you also consume the bones, for example sardines or anchovies), and seafood.

Milk is also good for our teeth. After consuming milk (or other dairy foods), oral acidity is reduced and saliva flow is stimulated. This reduces both tooth erosion and plaque formation. In the mouth, key minerals like calcium bind to the tooth enamel. Together, these factors mean stronger teeth and fewer cavities.

If you think that milk is fattening, you may have to think again. A number of epidemiological studies have shown that those with the highest intakes of calcium from dairy foods have lower weight for their height. In fact, dairy may help you to lose weight. Several controlled clinical trials have shown that having three servings of dairy a day assists in weight and fat loss when consumed as part of an lower-calorie diet. Dairy foods may also help to reduce weight gain, especially that seemingly inevitable middle-age spread. While discussions of the potential mechanisms involved have centered around calcium, when supplements are given in place of dairy foods the same results are not found (for a review of the evidence, see Zemel, 2005). While not all studies concur with these findings, they do suggest that there is something about dairy foods that goes beyond the calcium they provide.

Milk and dairy proteins have also been shown to lower blood pressure, and large-scale population studies have shown that those with the greatest milk and dairy food intake have the lowest blood pressure (Jauhianen and Korpela, 2007). Two studies in the U.S. have reported that dairy foods may protect against the development of type 2 diabetes and its precursor, insulin resistance syndrome (Lui et al, 2006; Choi et al, 2005).

All sounds good for milk so far, so why the controversy? Milk is more often than not among the first foods to go in popular detox diets and many alternative health practitioners in particular advise against consuming dairy. Many claim that milk increases mucus and nasal congestion, but scientific blind trials refute that this is the case. It may simply be that the creamy feel of milk in the mouth gives this impression. Nevertheless, many people report improvements in their condition when they avoid dairy foods so it is certainly worth a go if this affects you. Similarly, scientific research has failed to find any link between dairy foods and asthma. Be careful not to unnecessarily restrict your diet or your child's before taking known risk factors into account.

There is also some concern that a high dairy intake may increase the risk of two cancers:

1. Some studies, but not all, have found that high levels of galactose, a sugar released when lactose in milk is digested, may be damaging to the ovaries and raise the risk of ovarian cancer. However, reassuringly, a recent pooled analysis of studies showed no associations between any dairy food and ovarian cancer; although there was a slight increase in risk with the equivalent of three or more servings of milk a day, this was not statistically significant (Genkinger et al, 2006).

2. A Harvard study found that a high calcium intake (not necessarily from dairy) may be a potential risk factor for prostate cancer (Giovannucci et al, 2007).

These findings are by no means conclusive but they do merit taking a cautious approach. In fact, they confirm what can be said of many foods and nutrients, that some is good but more is not always better and may even be harmful.

There are two solid reasons to avoid milk: if you have an allergy or intolerance to milk or if you just don't like it. Allergies to milk (usually to the proteins present) are relatively uncommon and are usually found in children who, more often than not, grow out of their allergy. Far more common is milk intolerance, usually to the type of carbohydrate found in milk called lactose. In order to digest lactose, we need the enzyme lactase. Without it, lactose passes undigested into the colon where it is fermented by the resident bacteria. The symptoms manifest as abdominal pain, diarrhea, and excessive gas after eating lactose-containing food. Infants almost always produce lactase but, with the exception of Caucasians, most ethnic groups cease to produce it beyond childhood. This gives a physiological explanation as to why milk remains an important food for Caucasians, who originate from Europe where milk and dairy products are widely eaten, while most other cultures of the world do not drink milk. If you are lactose intolerant you may find you can tolerate yogurts containing live bacteria because these break down some of the lactose for you.

The bottom line is that because most of the world does not drink milk we can clearly live without it. But, if you like milk and milk products and have no problems digesting them, then these are fabulous nutrient- and protein-rich foods to choose. Therefore, we have ranked low-fat milk and natural yogurt as 5-star protein choices. These contain no sweeteners or flavors, can help suppress your appetite between meals making them great for snacks, provide the most readily absorbable form of calcium, and provide complete proteins, so they are particularly great for vegetarians and they are all low GI.

SEAFOOD

Like fish, most seafood provides good levels of omega-3 fats and is high in protein and low in fat, particularly saturated fat. All seafood is an excellent source of various micronutrients similar to fish, but is an even richer source of the minerals iron and zinc. Oysters and mussels score particularly well on this front because they are rich in both minerals. In fact, oysters are the richest food source of zinc, containing approximately 10 milligrams per oyster, while mussels have more than double the iron content of red meat. This makes them an excellent choice for those who wish to avoid red meat while still meeting requirements for these essential minerals. Other nutrients found in seafood include potassium, needed to maintain healthy blood pressure; phosphorus, for strong bones and teeth; and magnesium, needed for proper nerve and muscle function and heart health. For those who don't eat dairy products, oysters, prawns, and scallops become a valuable source of calcium.

Many people avoid seafood in the belief that it is high in cholesterol, but, in fact, this is only true for prawns, squid (calamari), and fish roe. We now know that diet affects our blood cholesterol levels and that cholesterol in our diet is far less important than the total amount of saturated fat. Soluble fiber in the diet also helps to prevent dietary cholesterol from being absorbed and so by eating these foods in the context of a plant-rich, high-fiber diet, they are far less likely to have a detrimental effect. Furthermore, given that these foods provide omega-3 fats and many other nutrients, they need not be avoided on the basis of their cholesterol level. Nevertheless, if you have been diagnosed with high cholesterol, it is prudent to limit your intake of prawns, squid, or fish roe to no more than once a week, but you can freely choose from the many other types of seafood on a more regular basis. For this reason, these three types of seafood don't quite make it to our 5-star category, but remain good choices.

Soy is a health food, right? So why is it not a 5-star food? Beneficial effects of soy have been reported in relation to heart disease, breast cancer, prostate cancer, menopausal symptoms, thyroid function, bone health, and even cognitive function. Yet, conversely, media reports and numerous websites claim exactly the opposite. Frightening headlines touting "the truth about soy" allege that soy is toxic to humans and causes numerous detrimental health effects including reproductive problems, an increased risk of breast and prostate cancers, decreased immune function, digestive problems, early menstrual periods in girls, and feminization in young boys. It's enough to turn you off your soy latte for life. But whom do we believe?

Soy is a legume that is fairly unique in the plant kingdom in that it provides all of the essential amino acids (the building blocks of protein) that humans need. In contrast, almost all other plant foods are missing or are low in one or more of these amino acids, meaning that vegetarians must consume a variety of plant foods to meet their protein requirements. For this reason, soy beans, tofu, tempeh, soy milk, and other soy foods have long been mainstays of vegetarian and vegan diets. But, on the whole, soy foods have not played a major role in the typical Western diet. In contrast, soy is regularly consumed by many Asians at all stages of life from weaning to old age. This difference in levels of soy consumption is what got the ball rolling in soy research. Scientists found that levels of heart disease and many cancers, including breast cancer, were far lower in these soy-eating Asian countries, compared to levels in the West. Numerous studies tried to identify what it was about soy that might be protective.

Research has centered on two aspects of soy: soy protein and compounds found in soy called isoflavones. Isoflavones are phytestrogens (meaning "plant estrogen") and are similar in structure to the hormone estrogen. These phytestrogens can act in two ways:

1. They can act like estrogen. This may be beneficial during menopause, for example, when natural estrogen levels drop. Theoretically, consuming enough phytestrogen-rich soy at this time can reduce menopausal symptoms.

2. They can block the action of estrogen. This is potentially beneficial in, for example, breast tissue where estrogen stimulates growth of both normal and cancerous cells. At least one of the isoflavones in soy, called genistein, has been shown in animal studies to inhibit the development of breast cancer.

Additionally, isoflavones have been shown to be powerful antioxidants and may in this way contribute to protection against diseases including cancer and heart disease.

SOY AND HEART DISEASE

In 1995, a report was published in the prestigious *New England Journal of Medicine* that concluded (on the basis of 38 controlled clinical trials) that soy protein significantly reduced blood cholesterol levels, particularly "bad" LDL-cholesterol and triglycerides (another blood fat linked to an increased risk of heart disease) (Anderson et al, 1995). On the back of this report, the U.S. Food and Drug Administration now allows food manufacturers to claim on the labels of low-fat foods containing at least 6.25 grams of soy protein that soy can help reduce the risk of heart disease. A more recent review of the evidence published in the journal *Circulation* suggests that this claim is rather premature (Sacks et al, 2006).

[TEXT CONTINUED]

It concludes that soy protein has only a very small effect on LDL-cholesterol, reducing it by a meager 3 percent or so, while having no effect on triglycerides or "good" cholesterol. Furthermore, the studies showing a beneficial reduction in cholesterol used large quantities of soy — approximately 50 grams a day. In reality, this equates to drinking about seven cups of soy milk or eating more than 20 ounces of tofu every day! You would have to be pretty dedicated to keep up this level of intake. Nevertheless, the authors did recognize that consuming soy foods in place of animal foods (high in saturated fat and cholesterol) should benefit the heart and overall health since soy foods are low in saturated fat, a source of healthy unsaturated fats, and rich in fiber and other nutrients. All this research is really telling us is that having soy milk instead of cow's milk and the odd tofu burger is not enough to bring down your cholesterol levels. But, choose the tofu burger over a regular burger, and replace the fattier cuts of meat in your diet with tofu or tempeh, and your heart will be thankful.

SOY AND CANCER

Some of the early studies comparing cancer rates across countries showed a benefit to soy consumption, and many soy and health food companies pounced on the results. However, the picture is far from clear, and a few worrying reports have emerged suggesting that con-centrated soy supplements in fact stimulated cancer growth in subjects with existing breast cancer. Of course, this often happens in nutrition research — scientists think they have isolated the important component of a food and try giving it as a supplement and lo and behold the effects are not the same. Try as we might, a good diet just cannot be packaged in a pill.

The American Cancer Society says that while soy-derived foods are an excellent source of protein, the evidence for the role of soy in reducing cancer risk, particularly the risk of breast cancer, is mixed. They recommend that for breast cancer survivors there are no harmful effects from soy when moderate amounts of it, no more than three servings a day, are consumed. However, they advise that breast cancer survivors avoid soy powders and isoflaven supple-ments because of the high levels of estrogen found in these products. For more information, visit www.cancer.org.

SOY AND MENOPAUSE

Many women have sworn that eating more soy foods during the menopausal years has helped reduce symptoms such as hot flashes and mood swings. However, the vast majority of studies have failed to confirm these anecdotal findings. Yet it is interesting to note that the reported incidence of hot flashes differs across countries with varying soy intakes. For example, while 70–80 percent of European women report hot flashes, only 18 percent and 14 percent do so in China and Singapore respectively. These differences are perhaps due to the way in which soy products are consumed, not as supplements but as key foods in an overall healthy diet.

SOY AND REPRODUCTIVE HEALTH

Reports of girls starting their menstrual cycle at an increasingly young age and the feminization of boys and men are among the more horrific of the claims made against soy. The basis for this is legitimate enough — that if infants are fed soy formula and young children consume soy in an increasing number of foods, they are exposed to the effect of an estrogen-like substance for a far longer period of time. Certainly infants in Asia are rarely given soy formula, but they are fed many soy foods from the age of weaning. These children have no ill effects on their reproductive systems and there seems to be little concern about soy foods.

[TEXT CONTINUED]

With respect to soy infant formula, a major study published in 2001 in the *Journal of the American Medical Association* followed more than 800 men and women who were fed soy formula as infants into adult life (Strom et al, 2001). They found no significant differences between this group and those fed a cow's milk formula, including any effects on the reproductive system. That said, there are those who seem to believe soy formula is healthier, and there is simply no basis for this.

The bottom line is that breast-feeding infants has indisputable advantages to bottle-feeding, but modified cow's milk formulas are a safe and effective alternative. Soy-based formulas were developed for use in infants allergic or intolerant to cow's milk, and therefore only consider using them if advised to do so by your doctor or health professional.

THE SOY BOTTOM LINE

While there seems to be little evidence to support the alarmist claims of the antisoy network, neither is there compelling evidence that soy is quite the health food some have cracked it up to be. The traditional Asian diet, rich in soy foods, has been shown to be a healthy diet that undoubtedly plays a role in their low rates of several chronic diseases including heart disease, obesity, and certain cancers. What they don't do is take concentrated soy or isoflavone supplements, nor do they consume a plethora of processed, packaged foods marketed as healthy just because they are made from soy, along with a diet too high in saturated fat and processed foods that is so typical of many Westerners. Traditional soy foods such as tofu, soy drinks made from whole soy beans, tempeh, and whole soy beans are healthy additions to your diet, particularly if they replace processed and fatty meats. But there appears to be nothing to be gained, and potentially much to lose, from trying to take the easy route and package soy in a pill.

FATS

WORLD'S HEALTHIEST FATS

☆ ☆ ☆ ☆ ☆

Avocado and Unrefined Avocado Oil

Camellia Tea Oil

Flaxseeds and Flaxseed Oil

Nuts and Seeds (including almonds, Brazil nuts, cashews, hazelnuts, nut spreads/butters, pecans, pine nuts, pistachios, sesame seeds and tahini [sesame butter], sunflower seeds, and walnuts)

Oily Fish (including salmon, trout, sardines, mackerel, herring, and mullet)

Olives and Unrefined Olive Oil

Seafood (including oysters, mussels, squid [calamari], and octopus)

For over two decades, health authorities around the world have recommended that we follow a low-fat diet. This was touted as the best way to lose weight and reduce your risk of heart disease. Many of us sat up and listened and did our best to comply. Food manufacturers did their part and produced a plethora of low-fat foods, including low-fat versions of many of our favorites which would otherwise be banished from a low-fat diet. We can now buy low-fat or reduced-fat cookies, cakes, milk, cheese, burgers, sausages, margarine, and even chocolate! The message that choosing these foods over their high-fat counterparts will do us good has been little questioned — until now.

While apparent fat intake has been declining in the U.S., and in most countries in the developed world, overweight and obesity rates continue to rise with alarming speed. Something is clearly going wrong. There are three alternative views of what that is:

1. Fat intakes are not really declining — it just appears that way from the methods used in dietary surveys. While many of us have made the switch to low-fat milk and choose lower fat products, we also consume more "hidden" fat in fast food, restaurant, and prepared meals, and in luxury treats such as ice cream, desserts, and candy.

2. Fat intakes have truly declined but what we are replacing the fat with is just as bad, if not worse, than what we were eating before. We eat more and more processed food that tends to provide the worst types of high-GI carbohydrates, low levels of nutrients and fiber and, despite their low fat content, these foods have a high energy density. In other words, they pack a lot of calories into each gram. While they are low fat, they are not low calorie.

3. The recommendations were wrong and lowering your fat intake does not in fact improve weight control over the long term.

There is evidence to support each of these three seemingly opposing views, and they may all be right or at least may all be contributing to the problem. The latest reports from large-scale studies in the U.S. have failed to show that reducing the fat intake of your diet in the long run has any beneficial outcome on being overweight, weight gain, heart disease, or cancer (Beresford et al, 2006; Howard et al, 2006a; Howard et al, 2006b; Prentice et al, 2006). However, what these studies have shown is that it is not the total amount of fat that is important, but the type of fat that you eat. In short, bad fats increase your risk of heart disease and certain other diseases while good fats lower the risk.

This explanation fits with all three of the views above. If view 1 is correct and we are simply eating our fat from different sources, then we are likely to be eating more of the bad fats and fewer of the good. If view 2 is correct, we are reducing our intake of all fats, including the good ones now known to reduce our risk of disease. And view 3 is directly backed up by this research, suggesting that recommendations to reduce total fat intake may be out of date.

This new research makes sense when we think of two of the healthiest known diets on earth: the Japanese diet, with a very low fat content of 20 percent; and the Mediterranean diet, with a relatively high fat intake of up to 40 percent. Both of these regions have low rates of heart disease which can't be explained by total fat intake. However, they do have several things in common, one of which is that both contain good levels of healthy fats and low levels of the bad fats. So what makes a fat good or bad?

THE BEST AND WORST OF FATS

THE BEST FATS WILL	THE WORST FATS WILL
predominately contain the good unsaturated fats	contain high levels of saturated and or trans fats
possibly be good sources of the essential omega-3 fats	raise blood levels of "bad" LDL-cholesterol
possibly be rich in other essential nutrients such as fat-soluble vitamins A, D, or E, and/or antioxidants	increase our risk of chronic disease including heart disease and certain cancers
increase blood levels of "good" HDL-cholesterol, while lowering "bad" LDL-cholesterol	may be stored more readily as body fat and burned less readily as fuel
reduce our risk of chronic disease including heart disease and certain cancers	be accompanied by nonfood additives such as preservatives, flavoring, and fat-replacers that have little or no nutritional value
possibly be burned more readily as fuel, helping us to lose body fat	

The different types of fats

Fats are made up of individual fatty acids that can be grouped into three main types — saturated, monounsaturated, and polyunsaturated. All fats contain a mixture of these three but will be predominantly of one type; for example, butter contains predominantly saturated fatty acids and therefore we tend to call butter a saturated fat.

The polyunsaturated fats can be further divided into the omega-6 and the omega-3 fats. The ratio between these two types of fats seems to be critical to health and, while in hunter-gatherer days man ate a ratio of close to 1 to 1, today we tend to eat far more omega-6 and not nearly enough omega-3, giving us a ratio closer to 14 to 1! The amount of each type of fat in common oils and fats is shown below.

TYPES OF FAT
IN COMMON FATS AND OILS

	PERCENT MONOUNSATURATED FAT	PERCENT POLYUNSATURATED FAT: OMEGA-3	PERCENT POLYUNSATURATED FAT: OMEGA-6	PERCENT SATURATED FAT
Butter fat	28	1	3	91
Canola oil	61	10	22	7
Coconut oil	7	0	2	91
Corn oil	29	1	57	13
Flaxseed oil	18	55	17	10
Lard	47	1	9	43
Olive oil	75	1	9	15
Palm oil	39	0	10	51
Peanut oil	48	0	33	19
Sunflower oil	16	1	71	12
Soybean oil	23	8	54	15
Safflower oil	14	0	76	10

Another type of fat is trans fat. Although very small amounts of trans fats do occur in natural foods, dietary intakes have dramatically increased due to our greater consumption of processed foods. Trans fats are produced during the chemical process called hydrogenation that turns a liquid oil into a solid. This was originally done in the production of margarine, but now hydrogenated oils are used widely in the commercial production of cookies, cakes, doughnuts, pastry, fast foods, and so on. In fact, many of today's margarines boast "virtually no trans fats" while consumers are unaware of the significant levels in some of these other foods.

So which are bad fats and which are good?

Primarily, this is based on how the fat affects blood LDL- and HDL-cholesterol levels. A high level of LDL-cholesterol can result in its absorption into the walls of the coronary arteries — this is part of the process of atherosclerosis which narrows the arteries and increases the risk of having a heart attack. A high level of HDL-cholesterol, on the other hand, is protective against heart disease since it is involved in transporting cholesterol back to the liver for elimination from the body. In general, therefore, the lowest risk of heart disease comes from low "bad" LDL-cholesterol and high "good" HDL-cholesterol levels in the blood.

BAD FATS

Saturated and trans fats both raise LDL-cholesterol levels and are therefore targeted as the fats we need to reduce in our diet. However, *trans fats are the worst of all*. While saturated fats raise good HDL-cholesterol levels as well as the bad LDL, trans fats *lower* good HDL-cholesterol while raising bad LDL. A key step to improving your health is to avoid these fats wherever possible. For this reason, we have ranked foods containing hydrogenated or partially hydrogenated oils as liabilities.

While most fat research has centered on heart disease and the effects of fats on blood cholesterol, there has started to be more interest on how fats may be metabolized differently and therefore contribute more or less to body fat stores.

While the research is in the early stages and is by no means conclusive, there is the suggestion that saturated fat may be stored more readily and burned as fuel less readily than unsaturated fat. In other words, is saturated fat more fattening than other fats? Since technically all fats contain the same calories per gram, this is a controversial idea, but given that this fits in nicely with the conclusions from the heart disease research, it can only compound the recommendations to reduce our intake of saturated fat.

GOOD FATS

Essentially, all unsaturated fats are good fats since they improve blood cholesterol levels, raising good HDL-cholesterol and reducing bad LDL-cholesterol. If you don't consume these fats and instead follow the traditional advice to eat a low-fat diet, you still reduce bad LDL-cholesterol but you also lower good HDL-cholesterol. This is undoubtedly part of the explanation as to why low-fat diets have produced such disappointing results in the long-term studies previously mentioned.

The omega-3 polyunsaturated fats deserve a special mention since they seem to be particularly important to health:

- Omega-3 fats can reduce your risk of cardiovascular disease in three ways: by "thinning" the blood, making it less likely that a clot will form and result in a heart attack; by protecting the heart from potentially fatal rhythm disturbances; and by improving the function of the blood vessels thus reducing blood pressure. Certainly for those with existing heart disease, consuming more omega-3 fats is arguably one of the most important nutritional changes you can make. A large European study found that in volunteers who had already had one heart attack, those who took an omega-3 supplement reduced their risk of dying from heart disease by 25 percent (GISSI-Prevenzione Investigators, 1999).

- Omega-3 fats have an anti-inflammatory effect on the body and are therefore also useful in treating (and possibly preventing) disorders that involve inflammation such as arthritis, inflammatory bowel disease and skin disorders including psoriasis, eczema, and acne.

- Omega-3 fats are known to be crucial for brain development and function. In fact, brain tissue from humans and animals has been shown to have very high levels of omega-3s. In babies and young children, omega-3s have been linked to development and IQ. Interestingly, breast milk contains these essential fats while formula milks do not, unless specifically fortified. Perhaps this explains some of the findings regarding childhood IQ and infant-feeding practices. However, we also know that omega-3s continue to be important for the brain into adulthood and have even been shown to be helpful in treating some forms of depression.

- Omega-3 fats have a role in eye function, and recent research suggests they may be protective against macular degeneration, a major cause of blindness worldwide.

- Omega-3 fats may be important for a strong immune system and may even protect against some forms of cancer.

- Omega-3 fats may even assist in promoting fat burning and improving body composition when combined with exercise. This was shown in a recent Australian study that reported a surprise result in which the combination of a fish oil supplement and exercise resulted in a 5 percent loss of body fat — an effect not seen in either treatment alone (Hill et al, 2007). Although more research is needed to back this up, it is an exciting result as it corresponds with an increased burning of fat during exercise, showing us that the type of fat, and not just the amount, you eat has an impact on your level of body fat.

In boosting your intake of omega-3 fats, it is important to make sure you are not simultaneously taking in too many omega-6 fats, since these will limit your ability to absorb and utilize the omega-3s. This is one reason why it is a good idea to use a monounsaturated fat, such as olive oil, for basic use rather than using a polyunsaturated fat such as sunflower oil.

How much omega-3?

How much omega-3 you need in your diet really depends on the results you want. If you have an inflammatory condition that may be helped by an increased amount of omega-3 you probably need to take a supplement, unless you are prepared to eat a lot of fish and seafood. However, be careful with supplements, as too much omega-3 can cause bleeding problems. Always make sure you tell your doctor about any supplements you take as, particularly if you are also on medications; these can interact with seemingly innocuous dietary supplements. For this reason, the FDA recommends that consumers not exceed more than a total of 3 grams per day, with no more than 2 grams per day from a dietary supplement. To give you an idea of how much fish you need to eat to achieve these targets, the table below shows the omega-3 content per 100 grams in descending order of typical fish and seafood. Swordfish is the resounding winner with over 1000 milligrams, so it is a real shame this fish is also one most likely to be contaminated with mercury and it is an unsustainable fish. Have it no more than once a week to be on the safe side.

OMEGA-3 CONTENT PER 100 GRAMS
OF SELECTED FISH AND SEAFOOD*

FISH	SEAFOOD
Swordfish 1059 milligrams	Krill (average of 2 varieties) 482 milligrams
Atlantic salmon 689 milligrams	Blue mussel 389 milligrams
Mackerel (average of 3 varieties) 461 milligrams	Squid 362 milligrams
Rainbow trout 309 milligrams	Pacific oyster 325 milligrams
Sardines (average of 2 varieties) 252 milligrams	Scallop 321 milligrams
Snapper 223 milligrams	Calamari 304 milligrams
John dory 188 milligrams	Baby octopus 214 milligrams
Yellowfin tuna 117 milligrams	Tiger prawn (average of 3 varieties) 114 milligrams
Cobia 113 milligrams	Rock lobster (average of 4 varieties) 106 milligrams

Nichols et al, 1998

It might look as though you need to eat fish every day to reach the recommended omega-3 intake, but remember you also get these fats in many other foods including meat, enriched eggs, flaxseed, canola, walnut, and mustard oils, leafy greens, and omega-3–enriched products (see "Types of Fat in Food" on page 80). To meet the target, most heart disease associations around the world recommend at least two fish meals a week, but think of this as the minimum. If you can, aim for three to five fish meals per week. This might sound like a lot, but remember that canned fish also counts, so fish meals can include a tuna sandwich. With a little thought and planning you can achieve an omega-3–rich diet.

TYPES OF FAT IN FOOD

GOOD FATS			BAD FATS	
MONOUNSATURATED FATS	**POLYUNSATURATED FATS**		**SATURATED FATS**	**TRANS FATS**
	omega-3s	omega-6s		
olive oil	oily fish, for example, salmon, trout, sardines, mackerel, and herring	seeds and seed oils including sunflower, safflower, and sesame (tahini)	butter	stick margarines (solid like butter)
canola oil	seafood, including mussels, oysters, calamari, and octopus	corn oil	visible fat on meat	commercially baked products including cookies, cakes, doughnuts, and pastries
peanuts, peanut oil, and peanut butter	flaxseed oil	soy bean oil	meat products, for example sausages, burgers, and salami	commercial, deep-fried foods, for example many fast foods
pecans	sesame seeds, tahini, and hummus	soft tub margarines made from the oils	palm oil	shortening
pistachios	walnuts and walnut oil	walnuts	whole milk	
cashews	meat from grass-fed animals	Brazil nuts	cheese	
hazelnuts	leafy green vegetables	pine nuts	lard	
almonds	omega-3 enriched eggs		coconut and coconut oil*	
macadamias	krill (small, shrimp-like crustaceans)			
	wakame (seaweed used widely in Japanese cooking)			

rich in saturated fats of medium-chain length, which are not cholesterol raising and have many potential benefits. See page 133 for more information.

— 101 Healthiest Foods —

BUTTER OR MARGARINE?

Life used to be simple. You spread butter on your bread, melted it over vegetables and used it in cooking. The biggest decision you had to make was which of a handful of brands to buy. Then new research discovered that saturated fat raises our cholesterol and increases our risk of heart disease. Over 65 percent of the fat in butter is saturated. Very quickly butter topped the "bad food" list and we searched for an alternative. Margarine, originally produced as a cheap spread, was suddenly promoted as the healthy choice and sales quickly overtook those for butter. But it all went wrong when scientists discovered that the chemical process used to turn an oil into a spread created a type of fat called trans fat that was even worse for us than saturated fat. Fast forward to today and the debate continues to rage as to which is the healthier choice — butter or margarine?

The use of butter can be traced as far back as 2000 B.C. and there are numerous references to the food in the Bible. What could be a more humble but delicious meal than bread and butter? In contrast, margarine was invented as a substitute for butter by a Frenchman in 1870, although only became widely popular during and after the war years. Today margarine sales far outweigh butter in most Western countries, largely due to the perceived health benefits. But can a modern, manufactured product, which goes against the nutrition purist's idea of eating food as close to nature as possible, really be healthier than the fat made from churning wholesome cow's milk? As passionate believers in eating "real" foods as much as possible, we have to confess to struggling with the idea that we can manufacture something that is better for us than a relatively simple food that has been made and consumed by native communities for thousands of years. But we'll give you the facts and you can make up your own mind.

From a nutritional point of view, there is no doubt of the winner. The saturated fat in butter is not good for us since it tends to raise "bad" LDL-cholesterol in blood, increasing our risk of heart disease. On the other hand, manufacturers of margarines responded quickly to the new information on trans fats and produced a new generation of margarines with little or none. If you read the labels of the vast majority of margarines on today's supermarket shelves, you'll be hard pressed to find any with a significant level of trans fats. The only ones to watch out for are harder stick varieties of margarine. Oils are liquid at room temperature; therefore, the harder the margarine is, the greater the likelihood the fats have been hydrogenated.

The fat in margarines comes predominately from the oils used to make the spread — canola, sunflower, olive, soy, and so on — and as a result they are high in healthy mono- and polyunsaturated fats. These fats have the ability to lower "bad" LDL-cholesterol. In fact a study of 46 families published in the Journal of the American Medical Association found that substituting margarine for butter successfully lowered blood cholesterol levels (Denke et al, 2000).

For butter lovers, take heart that butter does contain several essential nutrients — in particular the fat-soluble vitamins A, D, and E. Margarines are fortified with these nutrients to match the composition of butter. During our phase of obsession over reducing fat, these nutrients have been neglected. So if you love butter the answer is just don't have too much of it! Enjoy a little on your bread or a skim on your toast in the morning, but use healthier alternatives the rest of the time.

[TEXT CONTINUED]

Butter or margarine? We're going to play the devil's advocate and suggest neither. Butter is clearly not the best sort of fat for our heart health. Margarine is a modern invention and not a part of our ancestors' or native traditional diets around the world. After all, an olive oil margarine is not the same as a Mediterranean-style olive oil–based diet, and an omega-3–enriched margarine is not the same as a diet high in fish and seafood. So instead, brush your bread with olive oil, use a nut spread on toast, use mashed avocado in sandwiches, and cook with olive or other healthy oils.

A NOTE FOR CHEESE LOVERS

Cheese in general is an energy-dense food due to its high fat and low water content, and as such can contribute to becoming overweight if you indulge too much. This, together with the fact that it is a significant source of saturated fat, has earned it a bad name. However, there are many good attributes to cheese. It contains all of the essential amino acids and therefore is a great source of protein; it is one of the richest food sources of calcium; it provides other essential nutrients including vitamin A, phosphorus, and zinc; and when eaten at the end of a meal, cheese is good for your teeth by providing a pool of minerals that surround the tooth enamel.

The bottom line, therefore, is you can happily include cheese in your diet if you wish, but just watch how much. Ending a meal with an enormous cheese platter with crackers is not the best plan for health — save that for an occasional treat. Using strong cheese is generally a good idea as you'll tend to eat less, and you can also choose cheeses with a lower saturated-fat content for more regular use. The fat contents of the various cheeses are shown in the table below.

COMPARING THE TOTAL AND SATURATED FAT CONTENT IN 30 GRAMS OF DIFFERENT CHEESES

TYPE OF CHEESE	FAT (grams)	SATURATED FAT (grams)
cottage cheese	1.7	1.1
ricotta cheese	3.4	2.2
reduced-fat feta	4.3	2.8
goat cheese	4.7	3.1
light cream cheese	5.0	3.3
haloumi	5.1	3.3
mozzarella	6.6	4.2
reduced-fat cheddar	7.1	4.5
feta	7.0	4.6
Camembert	7.9	5.1
Brie	8.7	5.6
Swiss cheese	9.0	5.7
Parmesan	9.7	6.2
cream cheese	9.9	6.4
cheddar	10.1	6.5

CHOOSING THE RIGHT OIL

Further confusion over which oil to use occurs when you consider the extraction process and what you intend to do with the oil. The 5-star flaxseed oil can be downgraded to 1-star if you decide to use it in the deep-fat fryer!

The smoke point of oil is the temperature it can reach before it starts to break down. Heating an oil to the point of smoking will affect the taste and increase the risk of carcinogens in the cooked food. Most unrefined oils have a relatively low smoke point. Refined oils, on the other hand, have a much higher smoke point, but the methods used to refine them sometimes include numerous health-devaluing processes including bleaching, deodorizing, and de-gumming. Oils are generally refined unless otherwise stipulated on the bottle. The term "cold pressed" means the oil is naturally extracted using gentle, low-temperature extraction methods. "Extra virgin" is the name applied to the first batch of oil extracted directly from the fruit, nut, or seed. Oils that are predominantly polyunsaturated can easily become rancid when exposed to heat, light, and oxygen, and the processing methods may accelerate this transition. The price of the oil is therefore a good determinant of its quality. Cheaper oils are typically produced through a mass chemical-refining and extraction process, and while they have a high smoke point, they can ultimately be as bad for your health as cooking with lard. A safeguard from buying oil extracted and refined through a myriad of chemicals is to buy organic. For a product to receive organic certification, the entire process must be approved by the USDA's National Organic Program. Of all products used in the processing, 95 percent must be organic with the remaining 5 percent used from traditional natural ingredients free of synthetic flavors or chemicals.

AN EASY GUIDE TO SELECTING OILS

- Where no heat is required, the healthiest oils are cold pressed, extra virgin.

- Where moderate heat is required, select unrefined oils that can withstand the heat (see cooking guide on page 86).

- Where the highest cooking temperatures are required, select refined organic oils.

DO

- Stock a maximum of four oils at any one time.

- Buy smaller bottles and use them quickly.

- Store oils in the fridge or cool, dark cupboard.

- Buy oils in dark glass bottles.

- Check expiration date and throw out old oils that may be rancid.

[TEXT CONTINUED]

COOKING GUIDE FOR OILS
COOKING APPLICATION

UNREFINED	SMOKE POINT (°F)	COLD USE <225°F	LIGHT GRILLING AND GENTLE FRYING 225–350°F	MEDIUM FRYING AND BAKING 350–400°F	DEEP-FRY, STIR-FRY, BARBECUE >400°F	NOTES
Almond	221	●	●	●	●	Expensive oil for regular use — use in cold desserts or salad dressings. Use it quickly before it becomes rancid.
Avocado	250	●	●	●	●	Delicious and healthy, but expensive. Heavy flavored.
Camellia tea	195	●	●	●		Excellent-flavored, viscous oil for frying and baking.
Canola	107	●				Not a great choice when there are so many traditional, more flavorful oils available.
Corn	160	●	●	●		A soft, sweet, brightly colored oil.
Coconut	176	●	●	●		Used extensively in Asian cooking.

UNREFINED	SMOKE POINT (°F)	COLD USE <225°F	LIGHT GRILLING AND GENTLE FRYING 225–350°F	MEDIUM FRYING AND BAKING 350–400°F	DEEP-FRY, STIR-FRY, BARBECUE >400°F	NOTES
Flaxseed	107	●				Delicious, nutty-flavored oil for salad dressings. Is highly unstable and therefore must never be heated.
Hazelnut	221	●	●	●	●	Like all nut oils, an expensive oil for everyday use. Use it quickly before it becomes rancid.
Grapeseed	215	●	●	●		Light-flavored and suitable for most cooking and baking. Makes a good base for a salad dressing in which the oil carries other flavors rather than being the base for them.
Macadamia	198	●	●	●		Like all nut oils, an expensive oil for everyday use. Use it quickly before it becomes rancid.
Olive, cold-pressed	160	●	●			Best drizzled over salads and as replacement for butter with bread.
Olive, extra-virgin	205	●	●	●		Good all-purpose oil for moderate heat cooking.
Olive, virgin	215	●	●	●	●	Good all-purpose staple for everything.

World's Healthiest Fats ☆ ☆ ☆ ☆ ☆

AVOCADOS AND AVOCADO OIL

Avocados contain over 25 essential nutrients including potassium, magnesium, B-group vitamins, folate, and vitamin C. For a long time, avocados were on the dieter's list of "foods to avoid" due to their high fat content. Thankfully, we now know better, and the type of fat found in avocados is predominately healthy monounsaturated fat. The presence of fat also means that avocados are a source of the fat-soluble vitamin and important antioxidant vitamin E. Furthermore, if you add avocado to a salad or sandwich, the fat will then enable your body to absorb the carotenoids, and many other nutrients, found in the other plant foods. These are fat soluble and so if you only ever eat low-fat salads and dressings you absorb very few of these powerful antioxidants. Avocados contain several other disease-fighting phytochemicals including glutathione, involved in detoxification and antioxidant systems in the body; beta-sitosterol, which reduces blood cholesterol levels; and lutein, a carotenoid antioxidant thought to play an important role in eye health, preventing age-related macular degeneration, and in protecting the skin from sun damage.

Avocado oil may be new to you, but it is well worth seeking out. Look for one that is cold pressed and unrefined and you have an oil that preserves the nutrients and antioxidants found in the fat component of the raw fruit. The oil is very high in monounsaturated fat and very low in saturated fat making it pretty from a nutritional perspective. It also has the advantage of a higher smoke point than olive oil, making it an excellent choice for sautéing, stir-frying, and pan-frying.

CAMELLIA TEA OIL

A relatively uncommon oil in the U.S., yet one which has been used in Asian countries for thousands of years, is camellia tea oil, also known as tea seed oil (not to be confused with tea tree oil). The oil, extracted from the seeds of the camellia tea bush grown in the mountains of China has, like avocado oil, the advantage both in its refined and unrefined state of possessing a high smoke point, making it suitable for most cooking applications. It is said to be 97 percent digestible and used in traditional Chinese medicine to strengthen the spleen. With over 80 percent of its fat content from monounsaturated fat — even higher than olive oil — camellia tea oil is extremely stable and can assist in lowering high levels of "bad" LDL-cholesterol and reducing the risk of heart disease. It's another great source of the antioxidant vitamin E and provides the omega-9 family of fats, currently being researched for their effect on various inflammatory processes in the body. Refined camellia tea oil is organic and therefore free of any residual chemicals used during the extraction process. The oil has a unique smoky flavor and is delicious in salad dressings, stir-fries and even served with whole-grain sourdough bread.

NUTS AND SEEDS

As with avocados, nuts and seeds were once admonished, particularly as part of weight-control diets, due to their high fat and energy content. Yet research shows that not only do regular nut eaters tend to have lower body weights, they also have less cardiovascular disease.

Nuts and seeds provide a good plant source of protein, making them particularly beneficial additions to vegetarian diets. Nuts provide many other essential nutrients to benefit our overall health. They are good for our bones providing magnesium — 30 grams of Brazil nuts provide about a third of our daily needs — and small amounts of calcium, particularly almonds. They provide iron and zinc, two minerals that are often low in our diet, particularly if you don't eat meat. Cashews are the clear winners here: 30 grams of cashews provide women with 8 percent of their daily iron and 21 percent of their daily zinc needs (19 percent and 12 percent, respectively, for men). Nuts also provide a whole battery of B-group vitamins necessary to convert the food we eat into energy for the body, for healthy skin, hair, and nails, and to maintain healthy blood cells.

One large U.S. study found that eating a small handful of nuts (30 grams) on five or more days a week halved the risk of heart disease! Even those who ate nuts once a week had a lower rate of heart disease than those who rarely ate nuts (Fraser et al, 1992). Pecans, pistachios, cashews, almonds, and hazelnuts provide predominantly monounsaturated fat, while Brazil nuts, walnuts, pine nuts, and sunflower and sesame seeds are all rich in polyunsaturated fats. These fats have been shown to help lower "bad" LDL-cholesterol levels in the blood, while raising "good" HDL-cholesterol. There are even some super-healthy omega-3 fats in good quantities in pecans, walnuts, and hazelnuts. But it's not just the fat. Nuts provide a whole host of essential nutrients that benefit the heart. Nuts are fiber-rich and this undoubtedly contributes to their cholesterol-lowering effect. They also provide protein and, in particular, the amino acid arginine, known to be important in maintaining healthy blood flow through the arteries. Antioxidants are a major part of our defense against damaged, clogged arteries and nuts are full of them. These include vitamin E — almonds are a particularly good source of this vitamin with a small handful providing 80 percent of the daily needs of men and 100 percent those of women — as well as lesser known, but just as important, antioxidants including flavonoids, carotenoids, and phenolic compounds. In a study of total antioxidant power in different plant foods, walnuts ranked particularly high. Two to three Brazil nuts are all you need to meet your daily requirement for selenium. This mineral plays a vital antioxidant role in preventing cellular damage and is crucial for healthy immune and thyroid function.

Eating nuts may also help you to control your weight in two ways. First, nuts are very satiating and successfully curb our hunger and desire to eat. By eating nuts we avoid overeating other (probably less nutritious) foods. Second, nuts are an intact food containing lots of fiber — the body has to work hard to break down the individual cell walls to absorb and make use of the energy and nutrients. This, in turn, may mean that we are not 100 percent successful in completing the task and therefore fail to absorb all of the energy, particularly from fat, contained in the nut. In other words, we may be getting fewer calories and fat from nuts than predicted from the nutrient-composition data.

To get the most from these 5-star foods, steer clear of the salted, roasted varieties and the nut butters with added sugar, salt, other additives, and preservatives. Buy your nuts raw and unsalted — you can roast them yourself for a few minutes in a hot oven — and as natural, unadulterated butters. You'll find these in the health food section of your supermarket and they are delicious on toast instead of butter.

FLAXSEEDS AND FLAXSEED OIL

Flaxseeds (sometimes called linseeds) deserve a separate mention because they are fairly unique in that they provide a good plant source of omega-3 fats. They are not quite the same as the ones you find in oily fish and seafood; they are the shorter-chain versions from the same fat family and can be elongated in the body to produce the beneficial long-chain omega-3s. There is little doubt that regularly consuming fish and seafood is the best means of upping your omega-3 intake, but, for those who won't or can't, flaxseeds are the next best thing. Omega-3 fats tend to help reduce inflammatory reactions in the body and this may explain why some studies have shown flaxseeds to be helpful in reducing the painful symptoms of arthritis, gout, and inflammatory bowel disease such as Crohn's.

Flaxseeds are rich in both soluble and insoluble fiber. The soluble fiber helps to reduce cholesterol levels and slow the absorption of carbohydrates from other foods eaten at the same time, resulting in lower glucose and insulin responses. The insoluble fiber is beneficial for the digestive system, helping to keep you regular, providing a fuel source to beneficial bacteria, and keeping your colon healthy.

Flaxseeds also appear to have anti-cancer properties. They are rich in lignans, phytestrogens similar to those found in soy. These have been shown to reduce cancer risk, particularly cancer of the breast, prostate, and possibly the colon and skin.

To achieve a therapeutic effect from flaxseed, you need about 25 grams a day or a tablespoon of flaxseed oil. The seeds offer the most complete range of benefits and can be ground to form a flour or meal. The flour can be refrigerated for up to three days and sprinkled over cereal, used in low-fat yogurt or cottage cheese, or added to almost any baked item, including cookies, breads, muffins, or scones at 6–8 percent of the dry ingredients. Flaxseed oil has a very low smoke point and should therefore never be heated — use it in salad dressings or drizzle over your morning cereal.

OILY FISH

Oily fish are undoubtedly the best food source of omega-3 fats, and there is convincing evidence that eating more fish can reduce our risk of cardiovascular disease. If you have existing heart disease, eating more fish is possibly the most important nutritional change you can make. One large Italian trial found that people who had survived a heart attack could lower their risk of dying from a second attack by 25 percent by consuming 1 gram per day of omega-3 fats (GISSI-Prevenzione Investigators, 1999). In this trial, the participants were given an omega-3 supplement — to reach this level of intake from fish alone would mean eating a serving of oily fish every day. For the rest of us, we needn't consume this much to gain health benefits; the current recommendations are to include at least two servings per week of oily fish.

See page 80 for the omega-3 content of common fish and seafood.

OLIVES AND UNREFINED OLIVE OIL

Olives and olive oil provide the major source of fat in the traditional Mediterranean diet, and the low level of heart disease in this region is thought to be at least in part attributed to this. The fat is predominately monounsaturated, which is more stable than polyunsaturated fat, both as a food and once it's ingested and incorporated into cells in the body. It is therefore less susceptible to oxidation and bodily damage. As a food, the oil is less likely to go rancid and, once in the body, is thought to help prevent cancers by resisting the type of free-radical damage that instigates the cancer process. Olives and cold-pressed olive oil are also rich in phenol compounds that are natural antioxidants. They have been shown to have a number of desirable effects from helping to reduce skin damage from the sun to lowering blood-cholesterol levels, blood pressure, and the risk of heart disease (Covas et al, 2006). However, the phenol content of olive oil is not consistent, and many of the mass-market oils available in the supermarket have poor levels. There are differences between olive varieties and whether the olives are picked late or early in the season, but the major effects on phenol content are how the oil is processed and the length of time the oil is subsequently stored. Most of the standard olive oils have been refined — a process involving filtering, charcoal treatment, heating, and chemical treatment to adjust acidity — and this dramatically reduces the phenol content. According to the Olive Oil Source (www.oliveoilsource.com), unrefined, cold-pressed olive oil contains 50–80 parts-per-million phenols, while refined oil has only 5 parts-per-million. The longer the oil is stored, whether in storage tanks at the manufacturing plant or in the bottle in your pantry, the more phenols are slowly oxidized and used up. So in order to ensure you have an oil with a high antioxidant-phenol content, choose a high-quality extra-virgin olive oil that is from the current harvest season and that has been properly stored. The bottle should be a dark color to reduce exposure to light and the oil should be bought in small quantities to reduce storage time. You may have to look in a quality health food store or deli for the best choice. These contain as many as 5 milligrams of antioxidant phenols in every 10 grams of olive oil. Of course, this type of oil will be more expensive than the supermarket varieties, so keep it specifically for dressings and other cold uses. For cooking, a cheaper olive oil is fine, and, because of the effects of heat on extra-virgin cold-pressed oils (see section on cooking with oils page 85), you'll still get the good fats but not such high levels of phenols. Be aware that light olive oils are not lower in calories, but are more mild than other varieties for those who do not like a strong olive flavor. These oils are almost always refined, and, as a consequence, lack the wonderful antioxidants found in the more flavorful virgin oils.

SEAFOOD

While oily fish is more often credited for its omega-3 content, seafood can be equally rich. See page 79 to compare the omega-3 content of popular fish and seafood, and page 68 for general nutritional information on these nutrient-packed foods.

DRINKS

WORLD'S HEALTHIEST DRINKS

☆ ☆ ☆ ☆ ☆

Fresh Vegetable Juice

Herbal Tea

Rooibos Tea

Sparkling or Still Mineral Water

Tea (including black, green, white, and oolong)

Water

Drinks are often forgotten when it comes to making diet and lifestyle changes in the name of good health. In fact, the only common message we tend to hear is that we need to drink more water. This is certainly true for many, but given the vast array of drinks now available we really need to know more.

One of the problems with drinks is that they are very easily absorbed, giving us easy access to the calories they contain. This might sound like a good thing, but since most of us are watching our waistlines if not actively trying to reduce them, these easily absorbed calories are not of such a high quality. Furthermore, drinks bypass many of the appetite-feedback systems to the brain that work when we eat solid foods. In short, this means it is all too easy to knock back hundreds of extra calories without your body reducing your appetite and switching off your rumbling tummy. The result — you eat the same amount of food but add all those extra calories and wonder why you are gaining weight or failing to lose it.

But it's not all down to calories — there are many nutrients and phytochemicals to be found in the drinks we choose that can do us much benefit beyond providing simple hydration. Teas and vegetable juices are great examples. On the downside, drinks can be calorie-free yet be loaded with undesirable additives, flavorings, and sweeteners that have the potential to do much harm over the long term. So let's look beyond water and consider the other drinks that may be frequent indulgences or that might tempt us with confusing advertising and image.

TEA

Tea is the most commonly consumed beverage in the world after water. Its origins are in China where tea has been enjoyed for more than 4000 years. White, green, black, and oolong tea all come from the same camellia plant but undergo different processing to give them their characteristic flavors.

Essentially, the difference between green and black tea is that green tea undergoes less processing; it is simply the steamed and dried leaves of the plant, whereas, to make black tea, the leaves undergo an additional stage of oxidation before drying. This produces a darker, generally stronger color and flavor. White tea is a specialty of the Chinese province Fujian, is made from less-mature leaves than green tea, and is the least-processed tea. Oolong tea is a traditional Chinese tea, is semi-oxidized, and is somewhere in between black and green tea. If you don't like the slightly grassy taste of green tea, oolong may be for you.

All teas contain the potent antioxidants collectively called polyphenols. However, the level of processing affects the type of polyphenol present. White and green teas have a far higher quantity of catechins, shown in human and animal studies to have the potential to reduce the risk of heart disease and cancer. Green tea in particular has received a lot of positive press regarding its health benefits, some of which has been attributed to the catechin EGCG (epigallocatechin gallate) found in abundance in these less processed teas. However, other studies, including a direct comparison of green and black teas, have found no difference in total antioxidant capacity of different teas. It's just that the oxidation of the leaves to make black tea produces a different polyphenol group called theaflavins. Whether there are greater health benefits of one or other of these antioxidants is not really known. In fact, to say one tea is healthier than another seems to us to be splitting hairs. There is convincing evidence for the benefits of both green and black tea, the most commonly consumed, and so which one you choose to drink is up to you. Why not stock your pantry with different types to be sure of having the full range of tea antioxidants?

If you want a tea that is caffeine-free, you can choose form herbal teas or rooibos. These are not technically teas and should more correctly be called tisanes. Herbal teas are simply infusions made with herbs, flowers, fruit, roots, spices, or other parts of the plant. They do not therefore contain the same polyphenols as tea, nor confer the same health benefits. Also be aware that many of the health claims made on the packets of herbal teas are not proven and are dubious at best. Nevertheless, they are caffeine-free, calorie-free, and may have other healthful qualities such as promoting relaxation and aiding sleep. Rooibos comes from South Africa and is becoming increasingly popular. It does boast a high content of antioxidants and is both caffeine- and tannin-free. You brew it in the same way as black tea, but may want to leave it to steep a little longer to allow the full flavor to develop. In South Africa they usually add milk and sugar, but it is delicious without and is of course completely calorie-free when enjoyed in this way.

COFFEE

Coffee has been enjoyed for several hundred years and people always seem to be divided on whether or not it is good for us. Coffee has a mild stimulatory effect on the central nervous system, attributed almost entirely to the presence of caffeine. This tends to wake you up and make you feel more alert. But does it do us any harm? The evidence is not nearly as damning as you might think, and in fact coffee may even be doing us some good.

Caffeine can certainly make you anxious, but only at doses above about 600 mg of caffeine (Liebermann, 1992). Since a typical cup of coffee contains 80–140 mg of caffeine, that equates to consuming several cups. Normal intakes of caffeine, equivalent to two to three cups of coffee a day, have not been shown to increase anxiety in either healthy subjects or those with existing anxiety disorders. There is even some evidence to show that small amounts of caffeine can reduce anxiety. Caffeine has also been shown to increase several aspects of mental performance, including the ability to process new stimuli and increase the amount of information processed. So drinking coffee before that all-important presentation may well help to calm your nerves and improve your performance. There may even be a longer-term benefit. One study measured the cognitive function of over 1500 elderly men and women using 12 standard tests (Johnson-Kozlow et al, 2002). They found that the women with higher lifetime coffee consumption performed better in six of these tests.

Coffee may benefit the brain in other ways, too. Two studies — one retrospective case-control study (Maia & de Mendonca, 2002) and a prospective study involving more than 1500 Canadians (Lindsay, 2002) — have shown an inverse relationship between coffee consumption and Alzheimer's disease. Definitive conclusions cannot be drawn from only two studies, but these results have prompted further research. There is stronger evidence for a link between coffee and Parkinson's disease. A recent meta-analysis of 13 studies to meet the inclusion criteria demonstrated a 31 percent reduction in risk of developing Parkinson's in those who drank coffee compared to those who did not (Hernán et al, 2002). Without a doubt caffeine can affect sleep — both the time it takes you to fall asleep and the duration of sleep. But we are not all affected to the same degree. While some can drink coffee at bedtime without adverse effect, others find that having coffee at breakfast causes them to be tossing and turning that night.

This can partly be explained by habituation — the more coffee you drink, the less it affects you — but undoubtedly we all have an individual sensitivity to caffeine. For the majority of people, avoiding caffeine in the evening will prevent any unwanted effect on sleep.

Coffee has been shown to be beneficial in the treatment of asthma, probably by acting as a bronchodilator. As far back as the late 1800s, there are reports of caffeine being used to assist breathing in asthmatics. More recently, two large-scale population studies — one in Italy (Pagano et al, 1988) and the other in the U.S. (Schwartz & Weiss, 1992) — have found the risk of asthma to be almost 30 percent lower in coffee drinkers compared to non–coffee drinkers.

Much is made of the antioxidant content of tea, but coffee has in fact been shown to have a greater total antioxidant power than other beverages including green tea, black tea, herbal tea, or cocoa! The types of antioxidants present are, of course, different in each and

[TEXT CONTINUED]

it remains to be seen whether the characteristics of coffee really are protective. Epidemiological studies have failed to come to definitive conclusions about associations between coffee consumption and cardiovascular disease. In part, this has been due to confounding variables, where coffee drinking acts as a marker for some other lifestyle factor that is known to increase risk. Several studies have found that coffee increases blood levels of homocysteine. However, current opinion is divided as to whether homocysteine levels are in fact a risk factor. Either way, since the effect of coffee is relatively minor, it seems unlikely that there is any real effect on the risk of cardiovascular disease. As far as coffee consumption and cancer goes, there have been numerous case-control and panel studies to look for an association. In 2000, a review concluded that there was no evidence to suggest a link between moderate coffee consumption and cancer of any kind (Tavani & La Vecchia, 2000). It seems clear that for both cardiovascular disease and cancer prevention there are far more important dietary changes you can make.

The other big chronic disease affecting Americans is type 2 diabetes, and there may be good news for coffee lovers here. The famous Nurses Health Study reported early in 2006 that moderate consumption of both coffee and decaffeinated coffee may lower the risk of type 2 diabetes in younger and middle-aged women (van Dam et al, 2006). Caffeine could not clearly explain the effect, and researchers are now looking at other constituents of coffee for possible answers. A second study published the same year showed positive effects of coffee on several markers of glucose metabolism (Bidel et al, 2006). Coffee consumption was linked to lower blood glucose levels, both in the fasting and postprandial state, and lower insulin levels. Over time this could explain how coffee lowers diabetes risk. However, not all studies agree, and much more research is needed to draw firm conclusions.

You might think that the effects of coffee on the digestive system are unquestionable. But even here there is conflicting evidence. There is certainly evidence that coffee can exacerbate heartburn in some people, although not all. If you suffer regularly you could try switching to decaf as that seems to help some people — but, again, the published research gives conflicting results. Since decaf affects some people just as much as regular coffee, it seems likely that some other constituent of coffee is to blame. There is no evidence that coffee increases the risk of stomach ulcers or causes indigestion.

In conclusion, the potential hazards of coffee mean that we cannot class it as a 5-star drink choice, but the rarely talked about positives of this traditional drink really do make its bad reputation unjust. We have therefore listed coffee, perhaps rather controversially, as a good performer. Just exercise moderation over how much you drink. More to the point is the way you drink it. The American-style coffee bars with oversize cups, a vast range of syrupy, artificially flavored additives, and enormous quantities of milk and/or cream, can turn a relatively healthy, calorie-free drink into a nutritional nightmare. Keep it simple — skip the extras and choose skim milk.

TREATS

Although treats are at the top of the food pyramid model, and therefore should be a small part of a healthy diet, they are nevertheless an important part. The pleasure of eating and the sensory experience of consuming certain foods has always been an essential part of our relationship with food. The saddest thing we have ever heard in relation to food is a fitness instructor at one of our seminars in Sydney saying they would much prefer to take a pill to provide all the nutrition they need rather than have to eat real food. Let's hope we never, ever get to that point! Look at any culture or community around the world and food is a part of celebrating, socializing, commiserating, mourning — in fact almost every human event you can think of. Treats play a part in this and keep our relationship with food a healthy one. Guilt and eating have no business together — if you respect your body and enjoy your food, then treats, whatever they may be, you can healthily and happily have treats. The key is all in the quantity and quality of *all* foods in your diet.

Nevertheless, not all treats are equal; some have positive nutritional aspects and only a little potential damage, while others have nothing nutritional to offer (other than calories) and much that can do harm. You can afford to indulge more often in the former without compromising your health and well-being. To that end, we hope to guide you by relegating popular treats to their appropriate division. You'll notice there are no 5-star foods here because no treat is completely devoid of potential harm, but there are several 4-star performers that we can recommend. Enjoy!

Part 2:
Food Charts

WHAT'S WRONG WITH
<u>MOST DIETS?</u>

Given what you know now from the information on each food group, you can see that, when the hierarchy of our 5-star foods through to the 1-star foods is applied to various popular diets, these diets fail to give you everything you need and, overall, compromise your health.

In the typical diet, which has contributed to producing the fattest generation of all time, while there is a relatively good intake of vegetables (with perhaps a few fat-free, high-GI baked potatoes in there), there are far too many bad choices of carbohydrates and insufficient proteins. Low-fat cookies, crackers, cakes, and other high-energy, high-GI carbohydrates fill our cupboards and our stomachs. And, worst of all, many treats that we consider to be 1-star foods, since they have no nutritional value whatsoever, are considered okay.

The dieter following a high-protein plan may lose weight quickly — but at what cost? Diets high in 1-star fats, low in 5-star proteins, and lacking enough vegetables or fruits are likely to increase the risk of chronic disease such as heart disease and cancers. The lack of quality carbohydrates makes exercise difficult, and since these provide the best source of glucose to feed the brain, concentration and mental task performance are impaired. The lack of fiber in this diet means that constipation is a common problem and bowel health is seriously compromised. Furthermore, if you manage to lower your carb intake enough to force your body into what is known as a ketogenic state, your breath will smell and your head will ache. Yes, you will be burning fat but is it really worth it? We need to look beyond weight loss and consider our total health and vitality. Besides, could you eat like this forever? Neither could most people, according to much of the research to date. Such diets work in the short term, but over 12 months they perform no better than any other diet.

While it may be better than the previous two diets, the fitness junkie's diet is still lacking in some areas. Highly processed protein drinks and low-fat candies are common treats in this diet while fruits, because they provide carbohydrates, are frowned upon. No surprises here. The fast-food junkie's diet is worst of all — almost every food has a 1-star rating. We need say no more. The following pyramid below shows what to strive for. This is your winning nutritional pyramid. If, most of the time, you select from the 5-star and 4-star foods, you will look, feel, and perform at your very best.

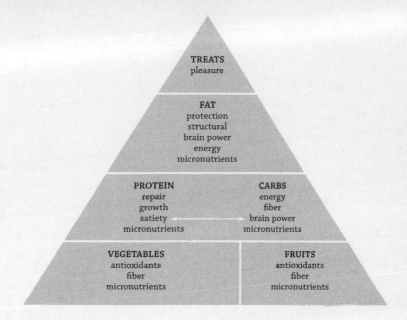

VEGETABLES

The table below summarizes the attributes of each vegetable, including key nutrients present, the GI where relevant, and any additional information of note.

VEGETABLE	Nutrient Summary
ASPARAGUS ☆ ☆ ☆ ☆ ☆	Very good source of dietary fiber, vitamin C, vitamin E, vitamin K, thiamin, riboflavin, niacin, vitamin B6, folate, iron, phosphorus, potassium, copper, and manganese. Good source of the antioxidant beta-carotene, which can also be converted to vitamin A in the body, and in two other carotenoid antioxidants, lutein and zeaxanthin. These promote eye health, reducing the risk of age-related macular degeneration and cataracts. Lutein may also play a role in preventing colon cancer. Good source of vitamin B5, calcium, magnesium, zinc, and selenium. Contains saponins, thought to reduce cholesterol levels and reduce the risk of heart disease, and rutin, an antioxidant involved in strengthening blood vessels.
THE CABBAGE FAMILY **(cruciferous veg/ brassicas)**	
ASIAN GREENS, INCLUDING BOK CHOY AND CHINESE CABBAGE ☆ ☆ ☆ ☆ ☆	Extremely rich in the antioxidant beta-carotene, which can be converted to vitamin A in the body. Very good source of vitamin C, vitamin K, riboflavin, vitamin B6, folate, calcium, iron, magnesium, potassium, and manganese. Good source of dietary fiber, thiamin, niacin, and phosphorus.

VEGETABLE	*Nutrient Summary*
BROCCOLI AND BROCCOLINI ☆ ☆ ☆ ☆ ☆	Rich in the antioxidant carotenoids lutein and zeaxanthin, which promote eye health, reducing the risk of age-related macular degeneration and cataracts. Lutein may also play a role in preventing colon cancer. Good source of the antioxidant beta-carotene, which can be converted to vitamin A in the body. Very good source of dietary fiber, vitamin C, vitamin K, vitamin B6, folate, potassium, and manganese. Good source of vitamin E, thiamin, riboflavin, vitamin B5, calcium, iron, magnesium, phosphorus, and selenium.
BRUSSELS SPROUTS ☆ ☆ ☆ ☆ ☆	Rich in the antioxidant carotenoids lutein and zeaxanthin, which promote eye health, reducing the risk of age-related macular degeneration and cataracts. Lutein may also play a role in preventing colon cancer. Good source of the antioxidant beta-carotene, which can be converted to vitamin A in the body. Very good source of dietary fiber, vitamin C, vitamin K, thiamin, vitamin B6, folate, potassium, and manganese. Good source of riboflavin, iron, magnesium, and phosphorus.
DARK GREEN CABBAGE, FOR EXAMPLE SAVOY ☆ ☆ ☆ ☆ ☆	Very good source of dietary fiber, vitamin C, vitamin K, vitamin B6, folate, magnesium, potassium, manganese, and the antioxidant beta-carotene, which can be converted to vitamin A in the body. Good source of thiamin, calcium, phosphorus, and copper.
RED CABBAGE ☆ ☆ ☆ ☆ ☆	Very good source of the antioxidant beta-carotene, which can be converted to vitamin A in the body. Very good source of dietary fiber, vitamin C, vitamin K, vitamin B6, potassium, and manganese. Good source of thiamin, riboflavin, folate, calcium, iron, and magnesium.

VEGETABLE	*Nutrient Summary*
BELL PEPPERS AND CHILI PEPPERS ☆ ☆ ☆ ☆ ☆	Rich in the antioxidant beta-carotene, which can be converted to vitamin A in the body. Very good source of dietary fiber, vitamin C, vitamin E, vitamin K, vitamin B6, potassium, and manganese. Good source of thiamin, riboflavin, niacin, folate, vitamin B5, and magnesium. Provides small amounts of lycopene, a member of the carotenoid family and a powerful antioxidant. Preliminary research suggests lycopene may play a role in the fight against cancer. One of the few food sources of a lesser-known carotenoid called beta-cryptoxanthin, which may reduce the risk of lung cancer, colon cancer, and rheumatoid arthritis. Chilies can boost your metabolism if you eat enough of them!
DARK GREEN LEAFY VEGETABLES	
CURLY KALE ☆ ☆ ☆ ☆ ☆	One of the best sources of the antioxidant carotenoids lutein and zeaxanthin. These promote eye health, reducing the risk of age-related macular degeneration and cataracts. Lutein is also thought to play a role in preventing colon cancer. Also rich in the antioxidant beta-carotene, which can be converted to vitamin A in the body. Very good source of vitamin C, vitamin K, vitamin B6, calcium, potassium, copper, and manganese. Good source of dietary fiber, thiamin, riboflavin, folate, iron, magnesium, and phosphorus.
ENDIVE ☆ ☆ ☆ ☆ ☆	Rich in the antioxidant beta-carotene, which can be converted to vitamin A in the body. Very good source of dietary fiber, vitamin C, vitamin K, thiamin, riboflavin, folate, vitamin B5, calcium, iron, potassium, zinc, copper, and manganese. Good source of vitamin E, magnesium, and phosphorus.

VEGETABLE	*Nutrient Summary*
ARUGULA ☆ ☆ ☆ ☆ ☆	Rich in the antioxidant beta-carotene, which can be converted to vitamin A in the body. Also a great source of two other antioxidant carotenoids, lutein and zeaxanthin. These promote eye health, reducing the risk of age-related macular degeneration and cataracts. Lutein is also thought to play a role in preventing colon cancer. Very good source of dietary fiber, vitamin C, vitamin K, folate, calcium, iron, magnesium, phosphorus, potassium, and manganese. Also has good levels of thiamin, riboflavin, vitamin B6, vitamin B5, zinc, and copper.
CHARD/ SWISS CHARD ☆ ☆ ☆ ☆ ☆	Extremely rich in the antioxidant carotenoids lutein and zeaxanthin. These promote eye health, reducing the risk of age-related macular degeneration and cataracts. Lutein is also thought to play a role in preventing colon cancer. Also a fabulous source of the better-known carotenoid beta-carotene, which, in addition to its antioxidant potential, can be converted to vitamin A in the body. Very good source of dietary fiber, vitamin C, vitamin E, vitamin K, riboflavin, vitamin B6, calcium, iron, magnesium, phosphorus, potassium, copper, and manganese. Good source of thiamin, folate, and zinc.
SPINACH ☆ ☆ ☆ ☆ ☆	Extremely rich in the antioxidant carotenoids lutein and zeaxanthin. These promote eye health, reducing the risk of age-related macular degeneration and cataracts. Lutein is also thought to play a role in preventing colon cancer. Also a fabulous source of the better-known carotenoid beta-carotene, which, in addition to its antioxidant potential, can be converted to vitamin A in the body. Very good source of dietary fiber, vitamin C, vitamin E, vitamin K, vitamin B6, thiamin, riboflavin, folate, calcium, iron, magnesium, phosphorus, potassium, copper, and manganese. Good source of niacin and zinc.

VEGETABLE	*Nutrient Summary*
WATERCRESS ☆ ☆ ☆ ☆ ☆	Great source of the antioxidant carotenoids lutein, zeaxanthin, and beta-carotene. The first two promote eye health, reducing the risk of age-related macular degeneration and cataracts. Lutein may also play a role in preventing colon cancer. Beta-carotene, in addition to its role as an antioxidant, can be converted to vitamin A in the body. Very good source of vitamin C, vitamin E, vitamin K, thiamin, riboflavin, vitamin B6, calcium, magnesium, phosphorus, potassium, and manganese. Good source of protein, folate, vitamin B5, and copper.
GLOBE ARTICHOKES ☆ ☆ ☆ ☆ ☆	Very good source of dietary fiber, vitamin C, vitamin K, folate, magnesium, copper, and manganese. Good source of vitamin B6, iron, phosphorus, and potassium. Also contains cynarin, thought to be important for liver health, and the antioxidant luteolin, which has anti-inflammatory properties and may be helpful in relieving symptoms of hay fever and other allergic reactions.
MUSHROOMS ☆ ☆ ☆ ☆ ☆	Very good source of vitamin D, thiamin, riboflavin, niacin, vitamin B6, vitamin B5, phosphorus, potassium, copper, and selenium. A good source of dietary fiber, protein, vitamin C, folate, iron, zinc, and manganese. Shiitake and other Asian varieties seem to be particularly rich in additional phytochemicals that may provide defense against cancer and other chronic diseases.

VEGETABLE	*Nutrient Summary*
THE ONION FAMILY (ALLIUMS)	
GARLIC, ONIONS, LEEKS, GREEN ONIONS, AND SHALLOTS ☆ ☆ ☆ ☆ ☆	Very good source of dietary fiber, vitamin C, vitamin K, folate, calcium, iron, potassium and manganese. Good source of thiamin, riboflavin, magnesium, phosphorus, and copper. Contain disease-fighting nutrients including sulphur compounds and antioxidants thought to be important in preventing cancer and heart disease. Shallots, green onions, and leeks are the more nutrient-dense of the onion family, while garlic has antibacterial properties. Onions and shallots contain fructo-oligosaccharides (FOS) that encourage the growth of beneficial bacteria in the colon.
PARSLEY ☆ ☆ ☆ ☆ ☆	Extremely rich in the antioxidant beta-carotene, which can be converted to vitamin A in the body. Good source of two other antioxidant carotenoids, lutein and zeaxanthin. These promote eye health, reducing the risk of age-related macular degeneration and cataracts. Lutein may also play a role in preventing colon cancer. Very good source of dietary fiber, vitamin C, vitamin K, folate, calcium, iron, magnesium, potassium, copper, and manganese. Good source of vitamin E, thiamin, riboflavin, niacin, vitamin B6, vitamin B5, phosphorus, and zinc.
PEAS, INCLUDING GREEN PEAS AND SUGAR SNAP/ SNOW PEAS ☆ ☆ ☆ ☆ ☆	Good source of the antioxidant carotenoids lutein and zeaxanthin. These promote eye health, reducing the risk of age-related macular degeneration and cataracts. Lutein may also play a role in preventing colon cancer. Peas contain small but useful levels of the more familiar antioxidant carotenoid beta-carotene, which can be converted to vitamin A in the body. A very good source of dietary fiber, vitamin C, vitamin K, thiamin, folate, iron, and manganese. A good source of riboflavin, vitamin B6, vitamin B5, magnesium, phosphorus, and potassium.

VEGETABLE	*Nutrient Summary*
TOMATOES ☆ ☆ ☆ ☆ ☆	Cooked tomatoes and tomato paste are particularly rich sources of lycopene, a carotenoid antioxidant that may be more powerful than vitamin C and was shown in preliminary research to provide protection from a number of cancers. Tomatoes also contain lutein and zeaxanthin, beta-carotene, and caffeic, ferulic, and chlorogenic acids — all thought to play roles in fighting cancer and other diseases. Very good source of dietary fiber, vitamin C, vitamin K, potassium, and manganese. Good source of vitamin E, thiamin, niacin, vitamin B6, folate, magnesium, phosphorus, and copper.
CARROTS ☆ ☆ ☆ ☆	Hard to beat for the antioxidant beta-carotene, which can form vitamin A in the body. Very good source of dietary fiber, vitamin C, vitamin K, and potassium. Good source of thiamin, niacin, vitamin B6, folate, and manganese.
CAULIFLOWER ☆ ☆ ☆ ☆	Very good source of dietary fiber, vitamin C, vitamin K, vitamin B6, folate, vitamin B5, potassium, and manganese. Good source of protein, thiamin, riboflavin, niacin, magnesium, and phosphorus.
SPROUTS AND BEAN SPROUTS ☆ ☆ ☆ ☆	Very good source of vitamin C, vitamin K, riboflavin, vitamin B6, folate, calcium, iron, magnesium, phosphorus, potassium, copper, and manganese. A good source of dietary fiber, vitamin E, thiamin, and niacin. Extremely rich in the antioxidant carotenoids beta-carotene, lutein, and zeaxanthin. The latter two promote good eye health by reducing the risk of age-related macular degeneration and cataracts. Lutein may also be important in preventing colon cancer. Beta-carotene, in addition to its role as an antioxidant, can be converted to vitamin A in the body.
FENNEL ☆ ☆ ☆ ☆	Very good source of dietary fiber, vitamin C, folate, potassium, and manganese. Also a good source of niacin, calcium, iron, magnesium, phosphorus, and copper.

VEGETABLE	*Nutrient Summary*
GINGER ☆ ☆ ☆ ☆	Can be an effective treatment for nausea, particularly motion sickness. Contains nutrients known to be anti-inflammatory. Early research shows promise for ginger in heart disease prevention by preventing blood clots and lowering cholesterol. Good source of vitamin C, magnesium, potassium, copper, and manganese.
GREEN BEANS, RUNNER BEANS ☆ ☆ ☆ ☆	Very good source of dietary fiber, vitamin A, vitamin C, vitamin K, folate, and manganese. Also a good source of thiamin, riboflavin, niacin, vitamin B6, calcium, iron, magnesium, phosphorus, potassium, and copper. Provides good amounts of the antioxidant carotenoids beta-carotene, lutein, and zeaxanthin. The latter two promote good eye health by reducing the risk of age-related macular degeneration and cataracts. Lutein may also be important in preventing colon cancer. Beta-carotene, in addition to its role as an antioxidant, can be converted to vitamin A in the body.
GREEN CABBAGE ☆ ☆ ☆ ☆	Very good source of vitamin A, vitamin C, vitamin K, riboflavin, vitamin B6, folate, calcium, iron, magnesium, potassium, and manganese. A good source of dietary fiber, protein, thiamin, niacin, and phosphorus.
OKRA ☆ ☆ ☆ ☆	Rich in dietary fiber and a very good source of vitamin C, vitamin K, thiamin, vitamin B6, folate, calcium, magnesium, phosphorus, potassium, and manganese. Good source of riboflavin, niacin, iron, zinc, and copper.
SUMMER SQUASH, INCLUDING ZUCCHINI ☆ ☆ ☆ ☆	Fiber rich and a very good source of vitamin C, vitamin K, riboflavin, vitamin B6, folate, magnesium, potassium, and manganese. Good source of thiamin, niacin, phosphorus, and copper.
SWEET POTATO ☆ ☆ ☆ ☆	The orange-colored varieties are rich in the antioxidant carotenoid beta-carotene, which can be converted to vitamin A in the body. All varieties provide good amounts of dietary fiber, vitamin B6, potassium, and manganese.

WINTER SQUASH, INCLUDING BUTTERNUT AND PUMPKIN ☆ ☆ ☆ ☆	Extremely rich in the lesser-known antioxidant carotenoid beta-cryptoxanthin, which may reduce the risk of lung cancer, colon cancer, and rheumatoid arthritis. Rich in beta-carotene which, in addition to its role as an antioxidant, can be used to form vitamin A in the body. Pumpkin also provides two other antioxidant carotenoids, lutein and zeaxanthin, shown to promote good eye health by reducing the risk of age-related macular degeneration and cataracts. Lutein may also be important in preventing colon cancer. All provide very good levels of vitamin C, potassium, riboflavin, and manganese and good amounts of dietary fiber, vitamin E, thiamin, niacin, vitamin B6, folate, calcium, and magnesium.
BAMBOO SHOOTS ☆ ☆ ☆	Very good source of vitamin B6, potassium, copper, and manganese. Good source of dietary fiber, protein, riboflavin, and zinc.
BEETS ☆ ☆ ☆	Very good source of folate and manganese. Good source of dietary fiber, vitamin C, magnesium, and potassium. Beet greens are in fact far more nutritious than the root, providing an excellent range of essential nutrients.
CELERIAC ☆ ☆ ☆	Very good source of vitamin C, vitamin K, phosphorus and potassium. Good source of dietary fiber, vitamin B6, magnesium, and manganese.
CELERY ☆ ☆ ☆	Very good source of dietary fiber, vitamin C, vitamin K, folate, potassium, and manganese. Also provides good levels of a range of carotenoid antioxidants which can form vitamin A in the body.
CUCUMBER ☆ ☆ ☆	Provides good levels of vitamin K and vitamin C and small amounts of various minerals.
CHICORY ☆ ☆ ☆	Very good source of dietary fiber, vitamin C, thiamin, folate, potassium, and manganese. Good source of vitamin B6, magnesium, phosphorus, and copper.

VEGETABLE	Nutrient Summary
PARSNIP ☆ ☆ ☆	Very good source of dietary fiber, vitamin C, vitamin K, folate, and manganese. Good source of potassium. Parsnips do have a high GI but you can ignore this since they have very few carbohydrates in a typical serving.
EGGPLANT ☆ ☆ ☆	Rich in dietary fiber and a very good source of folate, potassium, and manganese. Good source of vitamin C, vitamin K, thiamin, niacin, vitamin B6, vitamin B5, magnesium, phosphorus, and copper.
RADISH/ WHITE RADISH (DAIKONS) ☆ ☆ ☆	Fiber-rich and a good source of vitamin C, folate, potassium, riboflavin, vitamin B6, calcium, magnesium, copper, and manganese. White radish, or daikons, are the Asian variety.
SMALL, WAXY POTATOES ☆ ☆ ☆	These have a lower GI than large, floury potatoes and are therefore a better choice. However, aside from providing carbohydrate energy, potatoes are not particularly nutrient rich. They do provide good levels of vitamin C, but this is easily destroyed during storage and cooking. The skin is more nutrient rich than the flesh and provides good levels of fiber, vitamin B6, and potassium.
TARO ☆ ☆ ☆	Not so popular in the U.S. mainland, but a staple in many tropical regions of the world. A starchy vegetable that has a low GI providing a slow-burning energy source. Good source of dietary fiber, vitamin E, vitamin B6, potassium, and manganese. The leaves can also be eaten and are highly nutritious if you can find them.
TURNIP/ RUTABAGA ☆ ☆ ☆	Fiber-rich and provides reasonable levels of vitamin C, manganese, vitamin B6, folate, calcium, potassium, and copper.
YAMS ☆ ☆ ☆	High in carbohydrates but also low GI and therefore filling, providing long-lasting energy. Very good source of vitamin C. Good source of dietary fiber, vitamin B6, potassium, and manganese.

VEGETABLE	*Nutrient Summary*
LARGE, FLOURY POTATOES ☆ ☆	Very high GI and easy to overeat in all forms. These types of potatoes have been bred for a bland taste, white color, and large size. As a result, they are far removed from the original plant form and are, unfortunately, far less nutritious. They have some vitamin C and are a good carb source for recovery after strenuous exercise. For most people, however, there are far more nutritious choices to be had.
NONE ☆	None. All veggies have something to offer us, and the only concern would be in how they were handled, for example by deep-frying, overcooking, and processing.

FRESH FRUITS

The table below summarizes the attributes of each fruit, including key nutrients present, the GI where relevant, and any additional information of note.

FRESH FRUIT	Nutrient Summary
APRICOTS ☆ ☆ ☆ ☆ ☆	Good range of several carotenoids, particularly beta-carotene which, in addition to its antioxidant capacity, can also be used to form vitamin A in the body. Good source of niacin.
AVOCADOS ☆ ☆ ☆ ☆ ☆	Good source of vitamin K, niacin, and thiamin. Higher in energy than other fruits due to its high fat content — but it has the healthy fats that we want (see pages 76–80). The fat content also means that this fruit has excellent levels of fat-soluble vitamin E, which is itself a powerful antioxidant important in reducing the risk of heart disease. Great source of fiber.
BERRIES, INCLUDING BLUEBERRIES, BLACKBERRIES, CRANBERRIES, RASPBERRIES, AND STRAWBERRIES ☆ ☆ ☆ ☆ ☆	All berries are packed with disease-fighting, anti-aging potential and are hard to beat for antioxidant power, which comes primarily from the purple/red colored anthocyanins. High in fiber. All berries are very good sources of vitamin C, vitamin K, and manganese. In addition, blackberries contain good levels of vitamin E, folate, magnesium, potassium, and copper; raspberries contain magnesium; cranberries have vitamin E; and strawberries have folate and potassium. Wild blueberries, if you can find them, are even more antioxidant-rich. Be careful with cranberries — unfortunately the tart nature of these berries means we have to cook them and add sweetener. This can substantially reduce the nutrients and increase the energy density. However, they do have antimicrobial qualities that can be useful in preventing urinary tract infections. Beware of the juices, which can be very high in added sugar.

CITRUS FRUIT

GRAPEFRUIT ☆ ☆ ☆ ☆ ☆	Lacks the carotenoids of the pink varieties but remains a 5-star choice, providing good total antioxidant power and excellent vitamin C levels.
KUMQUAT ☆ ☆ ☆ ☆ ☆	The essential oils in the peel of citrus fruit contain phytochemicals that have demonstrated anti-cancer effects; for example, limonene increases the levels of liver enzymes involved in detoxifying carcinogens. Since we eat the whole fruit of the kumquat, this less-consumed citrus fruit may be particularly beneficial. Also a good source of thiamin. Kumquats are best stewed with a little natural sweetener such as apple juice concentrate or honey.
ORANGES ☆ ☆ ☆ ☆ ☆	Well known for their vitamin C content, oranges also contain a wide range of protective phytochemicals in the flesh, smaller levels in the juice, and, as with kumquats, in the peel. Try adding the zest of an orange to a dish or use an orange fruit spread that contains the peel. Also a good source of thiamin.
PINK GRAPEFRUIT ☆ ☆ ☆ ☆ ☆	Packs more nutrition than regular grapefruit thanks to the presence of the carotenoids that give them their pink color. These include beta-carotene, an antioxidant that can be used to form vitamin A in the body, and the powerful antioxidant lycopene, which is also found in tomatoes.
GUAVA ☆ ☆ ☆ ☆ ☆	The fruit with the highest vitamin-C content by a long shot! The carotenoids present give them their pink color. These include beta-carotene, an antioxidant that can be used to form vitamin A in the body, and the powerful antioxidant lycopene, which is also found in tomatoes. Good source of copper and manganese.
KIWIFRUIT ☆ ☆ ☆ ☆ ☆	Only guava contains more vitamin C! Very good source of vitamin K. Good source of vitamin E and copper.

FRESH FRUIT	*Nutrient Summary*
MANGO ☆ ☆ ☆ ☆ ☆	Rich in the carotenoid beta-carotene, an antioxidant that can be used to form vitamin A in the body. Also provides vitamin C, vitamin B6, and plenty of fiber.
PAPAYA ☆ ☆ ☆ ☆ ☆	Range of carotenoids present including beta-carotene, lutein, and zeaxanthin, which are important for eye health, and beta-crytoxanthin, a potent antioxidant linked to lower rates of certain cancers and rheumatoid arthritis. Great for vitamin C and folate and also provides good amounts of fiber and potassium.
PASSION FRUIT ☆ ☆ ☆ ☆ ☆	Wins the prize for the fruit with the most fiber, providing more than double any other fruit! Very good source of pro–vitamin-A compounds such that 100 grams of the fruit provides 25 percent of daily vitamin A needs. Rich in vitamin C.
PERSIMMONS ☆ ☆ ☆ ☆ ☆	Particularly rich in the carotenoid beta-cryptoxanthin, which has been shown to reduce the risk of lung cancer, colon cancer, and rheumatoid arthritis. Good levels of vitamin C and excellent for fiber and manganese.
POMEGRANATES ☆ ☆ ☆ ☆ ☆	This fruit has one of the highest antioxidant levels of all plants! Also provides good levels of vitamin C and fiber.
CANTALOUPE ☆ ☆ ☆ ☆ ☆	Particularly rich in beta-carotene, an antioxidant that can be used to form vitamin A in the body. High in the soluble fiber pectin. Good source of vitamin C.
APPLES ☆ ☆ ☆ ☆	Although not the broadest range or spectacularly high levels of individual nutrients, apples do contain an array of beneficial phytochemicals. Contain pectin, a soluble fiber that can help to reduce cholesterol lower the GI. Be sure to eat the skin, where many of the nutrients and the majority of the antioxidants are found.

BANANAS ☆ ☆ ☆ ☆	Very good source of several B-group vitamins, particularly vitamin B6 and riboflavin. Good source of manganese and potassium. Banned on low-carbohydrate diets due to their high carb content, but in fact a banana provides only a few grams more carbohydrates than an apple or pear and more vitamin C! At any rate, they have a low to moderate GI making them an ideal snack to tide you over to the next meal.
BLACK GRAPES ☆ ☆ ☆ ☆	Very good source of vitamin C and vitamin K. The purple color comes from a group of antioxidants called anthocyanins, which seem to have particular importance in maintaining healthy blood vessels and reducing inflammation.
CHERRIES ☆ ☆ ☆ ☆	The red color comes from a group of antioxidants called anthocyanins, which seem to have particular importance in maintaining healthy blood vessels and reducing inflammation. Good also for vitamin C and fiber.
GREEN GRAPES ☆ ☆ ☆	Very good source of vitamins C and K. Lacks the anthocyanins found in black grapes.
HONEYDEW MELON ☆ ☆ ☆	Not as nutritious as the cantaloupe but still a great vitamin C source. Also a good source of vitamin B6.
LYCHEES ☆ ☆ ☆	Rich in vitamin C and a good source of copper. Avoid those canned in syrup; buy them fresh when you can, or at least canned in unsweetened juice.
NECTARINES AND PEACHES ☆ ☆ ☆	Rich in vitamin C and provide fiber. Good source of niacin and potassium and provide beneficial amounts of a range of carotenoids.
PEARS ☆ ☆ ☆ ☆	Although pears can't boast spectacular levels of any nutrient or phytochemical, they do provide a good fiber and vitamin C boost for very few calories, making them a good choice for a sweet snack.
PINEAPPLE ☆ ☆ ☆ ☆	Rich in vitamin C and manganese. Good source of fiber, thiamin, vitamin B6, and copper.

FRESH FRUIT	*Nutrient Summary*
PLUMS ☆ ☆ ☆ ☆	Rich in vitamin C. Good source of vitamin K and fiber. The purple color comes from a group of antioxidants called anthocyanins, which appear to have particular importance in maintaining healthy blood vessels and reducing inflammation.
WATERMELON ☆ ☆ ☆ ☆	Particularly rich in the powerful antioxidant lycopene, also found in tomatoes, which gives it its pink color. Ignore the high GI of this fruit; the carbohydrate content per serving is very low, making the GI far less important. Fabulous low-calorie, nutrient-rich snack.
CANNED FRUIT IN NATURAL JUICE ☆ ☆ ☆	Less nutritious as the skin of the fruit is usually removed and certain nutrients, particularly those that are water-soluble, are lost during the canning process.
RHUBARB (STEWED WITH SUGAR) ☆ ☆ ☆	We think of rhubarb as a fruit, but it is in fact a vegetable. Raw, it packs a powerful nutritional punch, but unfortunately we need to cook it to make it edible, and this results in nutrient loss. You also have to add a sweetener and this increases the energy density.
CANNED FRUIT IN SYRUP ☆ ☆	The syrup substantially increases the energy content and adds a considerable amount of refined sugars. Also less nutritious than fresh fruit because the skin of the fruit is usually removed and certain nutrients, particularly those that are water-soluble, are lost during the canning process.
NONE ☆	All fruit has something to offer us, and the only concern would be in how they were handled, for example, by deep-frying, overcooking, and processing.

DRIED FRUITS

Note: The drying process results in a loss of some nutrients found in fresh fruit and are more energy dense than fresh which is why they fall into the good performing category rather than star. Prunes and apricots provide exceptional other quality benefits and are rated 5-star performers accordingly.

DRIED FRUIT	Nutrient Summary
APRICOTS ☆☆☆☆☆	Fabulous source of antioxidant carotenoids and make a good low-GI snack. Sulphur dioxide is used to prevent browning of the fruit and the growth of micro-organisms. This has been found to be safe at normal levels of intake but, if you are worried, look for organic produce and get used to the brown color — the taste is unaffected.
PRUNES ☆☆☆☆☆	Famous for their ability to treat constipation, probably due to the good fiber content and the presence of other compounds which stimulate the digestive system. The presence of unique phenols and beta-carotene gives prunes an impressive antioxidant power.
APPLES ☆☆☆	Reasonable levels of nutrients and a low GI make these a good snack choice.
CURRANTS ☆☆☆	Good for fiber and a plant source of iron.
DATES ☆☆☆	Good plant source of iron, but their high GI means they are not such a good choice as a snack. Use in small quantities as part of a meal or as a snack.
FIGS ☆☆☆	Highest for fiber of all dried fruits — 50 grams provides 24 percent of your recommended daily intake. Good nondairy source of calcium. However, the mid-range GI and higher energy density compared to fresh fruit reduces their ranking.

— 101 Healthiest Foods —

GOLDEN RAISINS ☆ ☆ ☆	Mid-range GI, therefore use as part of a meal or mixed with other fruit and/or nuts as a snack.
MANGOES ☆ ☆ ☆	Vitamin C is usually preserved in dried fruit. Although no data available for antioxidant power, the combination of vitamin C and carotenoids suggests that mango would rank well
PEACHES ☆ ☆ ☆	Reasonable levels of nutrients and a low GI make these a good snack choice.
PEARS ☆ ☆ ☆	Reasonable levels of nutrients and a low GI make these a good snack choice.
RAISINS ☆ ☆ ☆	Good levels of nutrients including iron and antioxidants. They have a mid-range GI, therefore use as part of a meal or mixed with other fruit and or nuts as a nutritious snack.
CRANBERRIES ☆ ☆	Unfortunately, most people find the natural tartness of cranberries unpalatable, and sugar is almost always added.
NONE ☆	All dried fruit has something to offer us, and the only concern would be in how they were handled, for example, by deep-frying, overcooking, and processing.

CARBOHYDRATES

The table below summarizes the attributes of each of the carbs including key nutrients present, the GI, processing factors, and any additional information of note.

CARBOHYDRATE	*Nutrient Summary*
BARLEY — POT AND PEARL ☆ ☆ ☆ ☆ ☆	Low GI, provides B-group vitamins, good plant source of iron and zinc, and good fiber levels. Can help to reduce blood cholesterol.
BEANS AND LENTILS (legumes)	
RED KIDNEY BEANS, CRANBERRY BEANS, LIMA BEANS, WHITE BEANS, CHICKPEAS, CANNELLINI BEANS, BUTTER BEANS, CANNED BEAN MIX, MUNG BEANS, ALL VARIETIES OF LENTILS ☆ ☆ ☆ ☆ ☆	Low GI and good source of plant protein, soluble fiber, antioxidants, several vitamins, including folate (cranberry beans are a particularly good source), and minerals including iron and zinc. Phytates present do reduce the absorption of these minerals, but this can be improved by consuming a source of vitamin C at the same time.
BREADS	
WHOLE-GRAIN SOURDOUGH ☆ ☆ ☆ ☆ ☆	Low GI, high fiber, and rich in nutrients. The dense, heavy nature makes it very filling and hard to overeat.
PUMPERNICKEL ☆ ☆ ☆ ☆ ☆	Made with whole-grain rye flour, this bread is low GI, very high fiber, and packed with nutrients including B-group vitamins and iron.

Note: *Soy beans are not included under legumes here because they provide very few carbohydrates. We have included them in the protein group, see page 51.*

CARBOHYDRATE *Nutrient Summary*

TRADITIONAL STONEGROUND ☆ ☆ ☆ ☆ ☆	Low GI due to traditional method of coarse grinding the flour. Look for varieties made with the whole grain to maximize nutrient intake.
WHOLE GRAIN ☆ ☆ ☆ ☆ ☆	Low GI, rich in fiber and source of many nutrients including B-group vitamins (note that whole grain is not the same as whole wheat; see text on breads, pages 45–46). Look out for breads made from the ancient grains spelt or Kamut®. Both claim to be better tolerated by those sensitive to modern, industrialized wheat and are nutritionally superior, boasting far higher protein and micronutrient contents. The downside is they do cost more.
BUCKWHEAT ☆ ☆ ☆ ☆ ☆	Provides all essential amino acids making this a great source of protein for vegetarian meals. Rich in fiber, low GI, and a good source of magnesium, copper, and manganese. Great alternative to rice and ideal for those with wheat or gluten intolerances.
BULGUR ☆ ☆ ☆ ☆ ☆	A fiber-rich, low-GI grain that is far more nutritious than rice. Great source of manganese, has good levels of magnesium, and provides significant amounts of several other nutrients.
CORN ☆ ☆ ☆ ☆ ☆	Low GI, high in fiber, and, particularly served on the cob, corn is an excellent choice in place of potatoes or rice because it is nutritious and easy to assign an appropriate portion size.
FREEKEH ☆ ☆ ☆ ☆ ☆	Higher in protein than regular wheat, low GI, very high in fiber, and nutrient rich. A good nondairy source of calcium. Available in most major supermarkets in the health food aisle.
NATURAL MUESLI ☆ ☆ ☆ ☆ ☆	Low GI, added nutrients from dried fruit, nuts, and seeds, high in fiber, provides healthy unsaturated fats. Great start to the day.

OATS (TRADITIONAL) ☆ ☆ ☆ ☆ ☆	Low GI and can help to reduce blood cholesterol, probably due to the good levels of soluble fiber present. High in manganese and provides good levels of thiamin, magnesium, and phosphorus. Buy the whole-grain, traditional variety and not the instant.
QUINOA ☆ ☆ ☆ ☆ ☆	A low GI and higher protein grain, packed with nutrients. High in manganese and a good source of copper, iron, magnesium, and phosphorus.
WHOLE-WHEAT PASTA ☆ ☆ ☆ ☆ ☆	Durum-wheat pasta has a low GI and has more protein than many other grain foods. Whole-wheat may take some getting used to but is well worth it because nutritionally it is far superior to white pasta and rich in fiber, B-group vitamins, iron, and zinc. Look out for pastas made from the ancient grains spelt or Kamut®. Both claim to be better tolerated by those sensitive to modern, industrialized wheat and are nutritionally superior, boasting far higher protein and micronutrient contents. The downside is they do cost more.
BRAN/HIGH-FIBER BREAKFAST CEREALS WITH LOW GI ☆ ☆ ☆ ☆	The high-fiber content is great for digestive health and keeping bowel movements regular — look for one with a low GI (for example, All Bran® varieties) and low added sugar.
BRAN/OAT MUFFINS WITH LOTS OF FRUIT ☆ ☆ ☆ ☆	High fiber and lots of nutrients. Good choice for a sweet treat.
BROWN RICE ☆ ☆ ☆ ☆	Nutritionally superior to white rice, providing more B-group vitamins and a good source of zinc and insoluble fiber, but since most have a high GI it doesn't quite make the 5-star category.
FAVA BEANS ☆ ☆ ☆ ☆	High GI but since there's not many carbohydrates per servings, this is not so important. Rates high for antioxidant content and overall good range of nutrients

FLAT BREAD ☆ ☆ ☆ ☆	Widely eaten throughout the world for centuries. Available in different grain varieties providing many nutrients. GI varies according to the variety: oat and white are both low; rye, barley, rice, and organic wheat are all moderate; and whole wheat and corn are high. However, since one slice contains about 14 grams of carbohydrates, about half that of a standard sandwich, the overall glycemic load is relatively low.
MULTI-GRAIN FRUITBREAD	Low GI because it replaces some of the flour with dried fruit. This also increases the nutrient content.
MULTI-GRAIN ENGLISH MUFFINS ☆ ☆ ☆ ☆	Low GI, high in fiber, and rich in nutrients from the whole grain.
OATCAKES ☆ ☆ ☆ ☆	Packed with nutritious oats but traditionally made using animal fat. Look for varieties with low saturated fat — those made with olive oil are now available.
CHAPATI ☆ ☆ ☆	Traditional Indian flat bread with a low GI. Lower carbohydrate load and less likely to be overeaten than naan bread.
COUSCOUS ☆ ☆ ☆	Mid-range GI, but a little goes a long way, making the carbohydrate load per serving relatively small.
BASMATI RICE ☆ ☆ ☆	Lower-GI rice variety. As with pasta, watch portion size if you're trying to lose body fat, but it's a great carbohydrate source for very active people. Brown rice is a better choice for nutrient content.
MILLET ☆ ☆ ☆	High GI but good plant source of iron, zinc, B-group vitamins, and useful for those following a wheat-free diet.
MUNG BEAN NOODLES ☆ ☆ ☆	Low GI and provides a good plant source of iron and small amounts of B-group vitamins.

NOODLES ☆ ☆ ☆	Most noodles have a low GI and are therefore a good source of slow-release energy. As with pasta, watch portion size and avoid those noodles that are fried before drying — read the ingredient list.
PASTA ☆ ☆ ☆	Low GI and has approximately double the protein of rice, but be careful with portion size if you are trying to lose body fat. Excellent carb source for the very active. Whole wheat is a better choice for nutrient content.
SEMOLINA ☆ ☆ ☆	Semolina is coarsely ground durum wheat before it is used to make pasta and couscous. It is relatively high in protein, has a low GI, and provides several nutrients including folate.
SOBA NOODLES ☆ ☆ ☆	Japanese noodles made from buckwheat flour. Although buckwheat is not related to wheat and is gluten-free, these may not be suitable for those with wheat or gluten intolerance as wheat flour is often added to help bind the noodles. Those noodles tested in Japan do, however, have a low GI, provide useful amounts of protein, and are a good source of manganese.
TORTILLAS ☆ ☆ ☆	Low GI and, although not nutrient rich, a good way to reduce overall carbohydrate load when served as a wrap in place of loaf bread. Unfortunately, commercial varieties have added preservatives to lengthen shelf life.
WHITE PITA BREAD ☆ ☆ ☆	Intermediate GI and less likely to be overeaten than more fluffy breads.
WHITE SOURDOUGH BREAD ☆ ☆ ☆	Traditional slow process used and acids present give a low GI. Lower nutrient and fiber count than whole grain, but the best white bread option.
BAGELS ☆ ☆	Very high GI and high carbohydrate load per serving. Advertised as low fat, but they are energy dense.

CRACKERS AND RICE CRACKERS ☆ ☆	Often found in a dieter's pantry because they're low-fat, but highly processed and high GI as a result. Rice crackers may have lower energy than potato chips, but while they may be almost fat free, they are not energy free.
DRIED RICE NOODLES ☆ ☆	High GI and few vitamins and minerals.
ENGLISH MUFFINS AND CRUMPETS ☆ ☆	Refined carbohydrates with a high GI. Easy to overeat. Low-fat but usually served with butter or margarine.
INSTANT OATS ☆ ☆	The additional processing of the oats increases the GI. Since the traditional varieties take only a few minutes to cook is there really any need for instant?
POLENTA ☆ ☆	GI of 68 so this only just avoids being categorized as high GI and is usually cooked with added undesirable fats. However, it does provide good levels of certain nutrients.
POTATOES ☆ ☆	Breeding of potatoes to produce fluffy, white produce has led to an extremely high GI. Lower GI varieties are small, waxy potatoes. The nutrients are found mostly in the skin so even less nutrition to be found in mashed and potato products.
LOW-FIBER, LOW-SUGAR PROCESSED BREAKFAST CEREALS ☆ ☆	Provides added nutrients, but high GI and heavily processed. Really, this is just like eating a processed, nutrient-poor food and taking a vitamin/mineral supplement at the same time.
PUFFED GRAINS ☆ ☆	Puffing grains significantly raises the GI, they are not very filling, and tend to not be rich in nutrients.
WHITE BREADS, INCLUDING BAGUETTES AND FOCACCIA ☆ ☆	Very high GI, made with refined carbohydrates stripped of the majority of the nutrients found in the whole grain. Very easy to overeat. Some concerns over residual chemicals from bleaching white flour.

WHITE RICE, INCLUDING JASMINE AND ARBORIO ☆ ☆	Very high GI and high carbohydrate load per serving, leading to large fluctuations in blood sugar and high insulin demand. Low in nutrients, as these are lost in the polishing of the grain. Great for athletes after training but not a good choice for most people.
WHOLE-WHEAT BREAD ☆ ☆	Confusing, as this sounds healthy, but not the same as whole grain. Whole-wheat breads are often made with mostly white flour with some whole wheat thrown in. More fiber than white but its GI is just as high.
COMMERCIAL CAKES, DOUGHNUTS, AND COOKIES ☆ ☆	Refined carbohydrates because they're made from flour and sugar mixed with the unhealthiest types of fat — saturated and hydrogenated vegetable oils. Preservatives, additives, and flavorings also usually added.
COMMERCIAL FRUIT MUFFINS ☆	So often considered a healthy choice, but most are really cakes made from white flour, sugar, and a small amount of fruit. To make matters worse, the serving size is usually enormous.
CROISSANTS ☆	Combination of refined carbohydrates with lots of the wrong kind of fats. High in saturated fat and can be significant source of trans fat.
PAPPADAMS ☆	Fried at high heat and no significant nutrients.
PROCESSED, LOW FIBER/ HIGH SUGAR BREAKFAST CEREALS AND BARS ☆	Often advertise their good vitamin and mineral content, but these ingredients are added. It's just the same as eating a bad diet and expecting a multivitamin and mineral pill to fill the gap. Almost all have a high GI and are high in added sugars.

PROTEINS

*Each food was assigned a rating based on its nutritional profile.
The criteria for the selection process were based on their ability
to maintain, support, and strengthen the body for optimal
performance. Consideration was given to the quality of the protein,
key nutrients, fats present, and processing factors.*

PROTEIN	*Nutrient Summary*
CHICKEN AND TURKEY BREAST — SKIN REMOVED ☆ ☆ ☆ ☆ ☆	Great source of protein that is low in both total and saturated fat. Organic costs more but assures you of a quality product that we believe is better for your heatlh and has a far superior taste. The next best option is to choose "free range" since neither organic nor free-range chickens have been fed antibiotics and they have access to an outside run (see pages 57–58 for more information).
EGGS — FREE RANGE OR ORGANIC ☆ ☆ ☆ ☆ ☆	Come pretty close to a complete food. Numerous vitamins and minerals (primarily in the yolk). Go for omega-3 enriched. Only 1½ grams saturated fat per egg, so unjustly labelled a "bad" food.
FISH — ESPECIALLY OILY ☆ ☆ ☆ ☆ ☆	Oily fish are the best source of omega-3 fats crucial for optimal health. All fish is low in saturated fat and contains all essential amino acids. Good source of iodine, iron, and zinc (see page 61 for information on mercury in fish).
GAME MEATS, FOR EXAMPLE VENISON ☆ ☆ ☆ ☆ ☆	Incredibly lean, very low in saturated fat, and provide omega-3 fats and all essential amino acids. Great for iron and zinc.

PROTEIN	*Nutrient Summary*
LEAN PORK ☆☆☆☆☆	A fabulous source of protein with very little total or saturated fat. Not as good as red meat for iron, but provides good levels of zinc and is a particularly good source of thiamin.
LEAN RED MEAT ☆☆☆☆☆	Low in saturated fats. Contains all essential amino acids. Excellent source of iron and zinc in particular. Look for grass-fed meats rather than grain-fed for lower fat and higher omega-3 levels.
LIVER ☆☆☆☆☆	Hard to beat for iron. Excellent source of vitamin A, vitamin C, riboflavin, niacin, vitamin B6, folate, vitamin B12, pantothenic acid, phosphorus, copper, and selenium. Good source of zinc. Contains all essential amino acids. Chicken liver has less total fat and less saturated fat than lamb. High in cholesterol, so limit intake if you have high blood cholesterol. Be aware that liver products such as pâté are usually very high in fat, much of it saturated from added butter or lard.
LOW-FAT MILK AND YOGURT ☆☆☆☆☆	Highest dietary source of calcium. Provides naturally low GI carbohydrates. Good source of phosphorus and B-group vitamins. Probiotic yogurts may help with digestive processes.
SEAFOOD (EXCLUDING PRAWNS, SQUID, AND FISH ROE) ☆☆☆☆☆	Good source of omega-3 fats and low in saturated fats. Fantastic levels of zinc and iron. Good source of potassium, phosphorus and magnesium.
CHEESES NATURALLY LOWER IN FAT, FOR EXAMPLE, RICOTTA AND COTTAGE ☆☆☆☆	Excellent source of calcium and provide all essential amino acids. Low-fat dairy foods have been shown in some studies to assist in weight loss, possibly due to high levels of the amino acid leucine present. No need to buy the diet versions, the small amount of fat in the regular varieties is fine as part of a healthy diet and they taste immeasurably better.

— 101 Healthiest Foods —

PROTEIN	*Nutrient Summary*
LEGUMES ☆ ☆ ☆ ☆	Listed as 5-star performers for carbohydrates, but are 4-star here because they lack one or more of the essential amino acids. Nevertheless, combined with other plant proteins, this is easily overcome and therefore legumes are an essential addition to a vegetarian diet. Good plant source of iron.
NATURAL YOGURT (FULL FAT) ☆ ☆ ☆ ☆	Contains the saturated fat found in whole milk, but excellent source of calcium and has no added sugar, additives, or flavors. Eaten in moderation, the fat is not a problem and does contain fat-soluble vitamins such as A and D.
PRAWNS, SQUID, AND FISH ROE ☆ ☆ ☆ ☆	All the benefits of other seafood but high in cholesterol. For most people this is not a problem, but if you have high blood cholesterol you should limit your intake of these foods to no more than once a week.
SMOKED FISH ☆ ☆ ☆ ☆	All the benefits of fish and but with a longer shelf life. Provides a convenient source of omega-3 fats. High sodium content of smoked fish prevents it making the 5-star category. Those with high blood pressure should limit intake. If your sodium intake is otherwise low, smoked fish can happily be a part of your diet.
SOY ☆ ☆ ☆ ☆	Plant source of protein that comes closest to matching the profile of amino acids from animal produce. Excellent for vegetarians. Low in saturated fat. High in antioxidants and phytoestrogens. High intake related to low levels of certain cancers in Asia, but concerns over potential increase in cancer risk with high phytoestrogen intake, particularly from soy supplements. Can reduce LDL-cholesterol levels and reduce risk of heart disease. Bottom line is choose natural soy foods such as tofu and not processed foods based on soy or supplements (see pages 69–71).

ORGANIC LOW-FAT SAUSAGES AND BURGER PATTIES ☆ ☆ ☆	The organic label means more than the source of the meat — it also means that no artificial flavors, additives, or preservatives are added. The shelf life will therefore be shorter than non-organic varieties, but the quality will be immeasurably higher. Look for those with a high meat content and low fat.
TEXTURED VEGETABLE PROTEIN (TVP) ☆ ☆ ☆	TVP is basically defatted soy flour that has been processed and dried to create a substance with a sponge-like texture which may be flavored to resemble meat. Used in products such as vegetarian sausages. Nutritionally, it provides a good source of plant protein with very little fat but, at the end of the day, it is a manufactured and processed product and as such is not a 4-star food in our book.
VEAL ☆ ☆ ☆	Veal is meat from a calf up to six months old. In Europe, the abysmal treatment of animals continues (despite aggressive lobbying from animal welfare groups) as this produces the very white meat prized particularly by French cuisine. Animals are individually penned to restrict movement and deprived of iron and sunshine. Although the American Veal Association has made strides to encourage that calves are raised humanely, there is no guarantee that all producers are heeding animal welfare issues and, for this reason, we cannot include veal as a 4-star food. Nutritionally it is very lean and low in saturated fat, and while not as high in iron as red meat, it is a good source of zinc and other nutrients.
CHICKEN THIGH, LEG, OR WING ☆ ☆	More fat, especially saturated fat, than breast meat. At home, remove the skin and any visible fat. Does contain more iron than breast meat.
DUCK AND GOOSE ☆ ☆	Fattier meats with a high proportion of saturated fat. You can significantly reduce this by removing the skin.

PROTEIN	*Nutrient Summary*
FATTY CUTS OF RED MEAT ☆ ☆	Significant source of saturated fat in Western diets. Watch out for grain-fed meats that may not have a visible layer of fat but have marbling, in which the fat is throughout the meat and impossible to remove.
FULL-FAT CHEESE ☆ ☆	Delicious to us cheese lovers but very high saturated fat content. You don't need to avoid it, just exercise moderation and enjoy a small serve. Undeniably great for calcium and good for your teeth when consumed at the end of a meal. Another dietary habit the French have gotten right!
FLAVORED YOGURTS (LOW AND FULL FAT) ☆ ☆	All have added sugar, and the low-fat versions are often the biggest culprits. They also use gums and other additives in an attempt to replace the creamy feel of full-fat yogurt. Full-fat, all-natural varieties are a better option but do contain more calories. Ideally, buy natural yogurt and add your own fruit purée.
WHOLE MILK ☆ ☆	Significant source of saturated fat if you drink a lot — a few regular lattes during the day adds up to a lot of milk. Kids under 2 years old need the extra nutrition from whole milk, but the rest of us benefit from skipping the fat.
REDUCED-FAT AND MANUFACTURED LOW-FAT CHEESE ☆ ☆	Less fat but also less taste than full-fat cheese. This means you're not really satisfied and either eat more or look for another food to eat as well. Choose the real thing, but exercise moderation.
COMMERCIAL BURGERS AND SAUSAGES ☆	Made from the cheapest cuts of meat, full of fat (especially saturated fat), and usually fried, adding to the risk of trans fats. Artificial additives, flavors, and preservatives are almost always added. Make your own at home using good-quality meat or choose organic low-fat versions instead.
CURED MEATS, FOR EXAMPLE PROSCIUTTO AND BACON ☆	High saturated fat, high sodium, and heavily processed.

PROTEIN	*Nutrient Summary*
DIET YOGURTS ☆	Artificial sweeteners may not have been proven to do us any harm but are clearly not real, natural food. Diet products leave us unsatisfied and usually we seek out more pleasurable food. Avoid anything labeled "diet."
SALAMI ☆	The solid fat you can see in lumps throughout the meat is saturated fat. Also high in sodium, and preservatives are commonly used.

FATS

The table below summarizes the attributes of each vegetable, including key nutrients present, the GI where relevant, and any additional information of note.

FAT	Nutrient Summary
ALMONDS ☆ ☆ ☆ ☆ ☆	Good source of calcium and protein, fiber rich, and good source of many micronutrients including folate, iron, and zinc.
AVOCADO AND UNREFINED AVOCADO OIL ☆ ☆ ☆ ☆ ☆	The fruit is fiber rich and provides many additional micronutrients including potassium, magnesium, folate, and vitamin C. Avocado oil has a very high smoke point and is therefore a great choice for cooking. It is quite expensive, but this is definitely a case for quality over quantity. Use it sparingly and a little will go a long way.
BRAZIL NUTS ☆ ☆ ☆ ☆ ☆	High in omega-6 fats. Compared to other nuts these come out top for magnesium, are good for calcium, and are a source of the antioxidant mineral selenium.
CASHEWS ☆ ☆ ☆ ☆ ☆	Good source of protein and folate. Particularly good source of iron and zinc compared to other nuts and fiber rich.
CAMELLIA TEA OIL ☆ ☆ ☆ ☆ ☆	We may be introducing you to this fabulous oil but it is definitely worth seeking out. It has a very high smoke point making it an excellent choice for higher-heat cooking in place of olive oil. Good source of vitamin E and other antioxidants.
FLAXSEEDS AND FLAXSEED OIL ☆ ☆ ☆ ☆ ☆	Flaxseeds are fairly unique in that they are one of the few plant sources rich in omega-3 fats. While not the long-chain omega-3s found in fish and seafood, these shorter-chain omega-3s are the next best thing. Flaxseed oil has a very low smoke point and therefore should never be used in cooking. Only use in salad dressings or over cereals. Delicious drizzled over porridge.

FAT	*Nutrient Summary*
HAZELNUTS ☆ ☆ ☆ ☆ ☆	Good source of protein and particularly rich in fiber compared to other nuts. Good source of many micronutrients including folate, iron, and zinc.
NUT SPREADS/ BUTTERS ☆ ☆ ☆ ☆ ☆	Rich in protein, fiber, and numerous micronutrients. Excellent alternative to butter or margarine on your toast and highly nutritious for both adults and children.
OILY FISH, INCLUDING SALMON, TROUT, SARDINES, MACKEREL, AND HERRING ☆ ☆ ☆ ☆ ☆	Provide the best source of the long-chain omega-3 oils, eicosapentaenoic acid (EPA) and docosahexaenoic acid (DHA), essential to health. Also listed as a 5-star protein (see pages 60–61).
OLIVES AND UNREFINED OLIVE OIL ☆ ☆ ☆ ☆ ☆	A mainstay of the Mediterranean diet. Antioxidant-rich. Associated with low levels of heart disease. Great for salad dressings and as basic oil for cooking (but not high-heat frying because the oil will burn).
PECANS ☆ ☆ ☆ ☆ ☆	Not as much protein as other nuts, but a good source of micronutrients including iron and zinc. Rich in fiber and antioxidants.
PINE NUTS ☆ ☆ ☆ ☆ ☆	High in omega-6 fats. Particularly good for zinc compared to other nuts and good source of protein, fiber and many micronutrients including folate and iron.
PISTACHIOS ☆ ☆ ☆ ☆ ☆	Good source of protein and more than five times the vitamin A of other nuts. Good source of folate, iron, and zinc.
SEAFOOD, INCLUDING OYSTERS, MUSSELS, SQUID, CALAMARI, AND OCTOPUS ☆ ☆ ☆ ☆ ☆	These foods are low in overall fat levels, but we include them here as they do provide good levels of the long-chain omega-3 oils (EPA and DHA) essential to health. Excellent sources of many micronutrients including iron and zinc. Also listed as a 5-star protein (see page 68).

FAT	*Nutrient Summary*
SESAME SEEDS AND TAHINI (SESAME BUTTER) ☆ ☆ ☆ ☆ ☆	High in omega-6 fats, so watch total quantity to balance with omega-3s. Good source of iron, zinc, folate, protein, and fiber. Tahini is particularly good for calcium.
SUNFLOWER SEEDS ☆ ☆ ☆ ☆ ☆	High in omega-6 fats, but you are likely to consume less than you will with sunflower oil. Good source of iron, zinc, folate, protein, fiber, and calcium.
WALNUTS ☆ ☆ ☆ ☆ ☆	High in omega-6 fats. Good source of protein, fiber, and many of the micronutrients found in other nuts including folate, zinc, and iron.
COCONUTS AND COCONUT OIL ☆ ☆ ☆ ☆	Coconuts have had a bad reputation, primarily because the fat they contain is highly saturated. However, these fats are not the same as those found in animal foods. The majority are medium-chain triglycerides (MCTs) and do not raise cholesterol levels. In fact MCTs are readily burned as fuel, leading many to suggest that coconuts may help with weight control when used in place of other fats in the diet. Coconuts also possess antiviral, antibacterial, and antifungal properties and are used medicinally in many parts of the world. Many people consider coconuts to be a highly nutritious health food while others continue to be skeptical. We therefore reserve 5-star status until further research strengthens the evidence, but as a natural, minimally processed food that has been eaten for thousands of years we give it 4 stars.
MACADAMIAS ☆ ☆ ☆ ☆	Don't quite make the 5-star category because, compared to other nuts, macadamias have less iron, zinc, and other micronutrients, less protein and more total fat, saturated fat, and calories per serving. Nevertheless, they provide healthy fat and are a good source of fiber giving them 4-star qualities.

PEANUTS, PEANUT BUTTER, AND UNREFINED PEANUT OIL ☆ ☆ ☆ ☆	The predominant fat in peanuts is healthy monoun-saturated fat. Peanuts and peanut butter are rich in fiber, a good source of B-group vitamins, and a source of iron and zinc. However, peanuts don't make it to our 5-star category as they are heavily over-produced and over-processed by the food industry. This is of concern with the rising incidence of peanut allergies. There is also some concern that, because peanuts grow in the ground, they absorb a far greater level of pesticides and other toxins than tree-nuts do. You can find organic peanuts and oil in good health food shops to eliminate this problem. Unrefined oil is not always easy to find because most is bulk-produced and refined for high-heat cooking. Otherwise, at least choose raw, unsalted nuts and peanut butter with no added sugar or salt, and aim to broaden your tastes to include other nuts.
UNREFINED GRAPESEED OIL ☆ ☆ ☆	Main fat is polyunsaturated omega-6 fat, so this is a 3-star rather than a 4-star performer. This oil does have a high smoke point and can therefore be useful for high-heat cooking.
UNREFINED SESAME OIL ☆ ☆ ☆	Main fat is polyunsaturated omega-6 fat, so this is a 3-star rather than a 4-star performer. But in small quantities it adds a delicious flavor to stir-fries and salad dressings.
UNREFINED SUNFLOWER OIL AND SAFFLOWER OIL ☆ ☆ ☆	Main fat is polyunsaturated omega-6 fat, so this is a 3-star rather than a 4-star performer, but is rich in the main fat-soluble antioxidant vitamin E.
WHOLE-EGG, FRESH MAYONNAISE ☆ ☆ ☆	Look for one made with olive oil, whole eggs, vinegar, and a simple ingredient list of only real foods with no preservatives, additives, or other non-food items.

FAT	*Nutrient Summary*
BUTTER ☆ ☆	Butter fat is about 70 percent saturated and therefore not a good fat to use regularly in your diet. However, butter does have some positive attributes. It is an excellent source of the fat-soluble vitamins A and D. It is also far less processed than margarines. When you really feel like spreading some on delicious bread or a special recipe calls for using butter, go ahead and enjoy — just don't make it a regular habit.
CANOLA OIL ☆ ☆	We have our reservations about this oil, not because of the numerous scare tactics employed by dubious websites — there is no evidence to support any of these claims (see page 85) — but simply because it is manufactured to meet a demand for a stable healthy oil to be used by the food industry (olive oil is too expensive and cannot be used for all cooking applications). As such, it is refined and processed in order to be heat stable for cooking. However, it is predominantly healthy monounsaturated fat and as such it is not a bad choice for cooking. We simply cannot include it in the same category as the many wonderful unrefined plant oils available.
CORN OIL ☆ ☆	Main fat is polyunsaturated omega-6 fat and it is low in saturates. However, this is a highly processed, refined oil extracted using modern high-pressure techniques, with no real evidence of its long-term effect on health.
FULL-FAT DAIRY PRODUCTS ☆ ☆	A significant source of saturated fat in many people's diets and an easy one to cut down on; simply choose low-fat milks and yogurts for everyday use. The exception is cheese — there are some good cheeses that are naturally lower in fat (check out page 83), but most manufactured low-fat cheese is also low on flavor. Go for the real thing but use it sparingly. Full-fat dairy foods do provide excellent levels of calcium and the fat-soluble vitamins A and D. Studies have also shown that cheese has a far smaller effect than butter on raising blood cholesterol. All in all, a little of these foods will do no harm, but keep the emphasis on "little."

FAT	Nutrient Summary
MONOUNSATURATED MARGARINES, FOR EXAMPLE OLIVE OIL SPREAD ☆ ☆	Olive oil spread is not the same as olive oil. While better than the polyunsaturated margarines since the major fat is the more neutral monounsaturated type, these are still highly processed products. If you love butter and find it hard to cut down, switching to one of these spreads is a move in the right direction, but far better to change how you eat to avoid needing a spread at all (see pages 81–82).
PLANT-STEROL MARGARINES ☆ ☆	Plant sterols bind cholesterol in the digestive system, carrying it out the other end instead of being absorbed. Eat enough of it and there is no doubt that a plant sterol margarine can significantly reduce your blood cholesterol levels, which then reduces the chances that you will need cholesterol-lowering medication. However, these are still processed margarines at the end of the day, and like all other margarines we cannot recommend them as 5-star foods. A major problem with them is that you must eat enough of the margarine for it to have any effect. If you have high cholesterol, you may choose to give these margarines a shot. But we think you are far better off changing your overall diet for long-term good health.
REFINED OILS ☆ ☆	High pressure and high temperatures are used to extract the oil, which is then refined using solvents, traces of which remain in the oil. Bleaching and de-gumming are often further treatments used, and both involve high temperature and/or chemicals. While there is no clear evidence that this is harmful unless trans fats are produced, the safety of these oils is questionable. Spend a little more for a quality cold-pressed oil.

FAT	*Nutrient Summary*
RICE BRAN OIL ☆ ☆	Gaining in popularity, this oil is extracted from the outer hull of rice grains. It contains a form of vitamin E that has been shown in some studies to lower cholesterol and be a powerful antioxidant. The fat profile is similar to peanut oil, with the main fat being monounsaturated. However, the extraction method used involves high heat and chemical solvents, therefore we question the healthiness of the end product. It is certainly cheap, but in the oil world price usually determines quality. The bottom line is this is a new oil without a lot of research about it.
ROASTED, SALTED NUTS, INCLUDING PEANUTS ☆ ☆	While nuts and seeds are generally a healthy addition to your diet, they are not when they are roasted in oil and heavily coated with salt. For healthy blood pressure we need more potassium and less sodium (salt).
SOY BEAN OIL ☆ ☆	Main fat is polyunsaturated omega-6 fat and it is low in saturates. But not an oil with a long history of use and can only be produced using modern high-pressure extraction techniques. Widely used by the food industry and often hydrogenated for use in margarines and other food products — avoid these products. Note: In our overall diet, we want to ensure we don't allow the polyunsaturated omega-6 fats to dominate over the omega-3s. A balance of the two fat types is crucial. Oils are the pure fat extracted from the nut or seed and are therefore a far more significant source of the fat than eating the whole food. For this reason we don't include omega-6–rich oils in our 5-star choices because a better choice is a neutral monounsaturated fat or oil that provides omega-3s. However, nuts and seeds that contain omega-6s have other nutritional attributes, and the total amount of fat you get from eating the whole food is far less, therefore most of these are included as 5-star choices.

COMMERCIALLY BAKED PRODUCTS LIKE DOUGHNUTS, CAKES, PASTRIES, AND COOKIES	Let's face it, most of us love a sweet treat and we certainly don't mean to banish your favorites to the "never" category. You can have your cake and eat it too so long as you choose the right cake. Commercially produced products are likely to use the cheapest ingredients, and that means the cheapest, least nutritious fats. These products are high in saturated fat, can have significant levels of trans fat, and are energy dense and nutrient poor. See pages 148–49 for delicious and nutritious sweet treats to opt for instead.
COMMERCIALLY DEEP-FRIED FOOD AND FAST FOOD	A major source of the worst kind of fat — trans fat. Caused by repeatedly heating oils to a high temperature which changes the physical structure of the fat. These products tend to be high in total fat, and energy dense but nutrient poor. Need we say more?
COMMERCIAL MAYONNAISE	Read the ingredients list to see whether it seems like a healthy choice or not. Commercial mayonnaise has preservatives, additives, and flavorings added and is usually based on processed egg substitute and undesirable oils. A far better choice is a fresh mayonnaise found in the refrigerated section that lists only real food ingredients. It's even better to make your own using olive oil and omega-3–rich, free-range eggs.
LARD ☆	You can still get lard in the supermarket so someone is still buying it. Don't! This is pure animal fat (100 percent fat compared to 80 percent fat in butter). It is extremely high in saturated fat and cholesterol and doesn't even provide good quantities of fat-soluble vitamins like butter does. We will concede, however, that lard is preferable to using a heavily processed and refined plant fat for use in pastry making and certain other cooking applications — in these instances, occasional consumption will not harm you.

FAT	*Nutrient Summary*
LOW- AND REDUCED-FAT SPREADS	It might surprise you that we think these are dreadful while most people assume these are healthy choices. However, these are highly processed, manufactured products that give you a false sense of security. Research has shown that we tend to use more spread if we're told it is low-fat than if we're told it is the full-fat original product. The ingredient list should be enough to put you off. Skip these spreads and instead use good-quality healthy fats in moderation.
PALM OIL ☆	This fat is often assumed to be healthy because it is a plant fat, and it may be labelled as simply vegetable fat. However, it is one of the few plant fats to be extremely high in saturated fat. This makes it a stable fat and therefore it's often favored in food production. Look for it in ingredient lists of pre-prepared and packaged foods, and if the oil is simply listed as vegetable oil assume it is palm oil and avoid it.
POLYUNSATURATED MARGARINES	These are usually based on sunflower or safflower oil and are marketed as a healthy choice. However, as with low-fat spreads, these are highly processed products and, let's face it, sunflower margarine is not the same as sunflower oil and a far cry from eating the whole sunflower seed.
SALAD DRESSING (CREAMY) ☆	As with commercial mayonnaise, read the ingredient list for reasons not to consume this food product. Making your own delicious and nutritious salad dressing is neither difficult nor time-consuming when you know how.
SHORTENING ☆	Sometimes this is made from animal fat, but more often it is hydrogenated vegetable fat. As such it contains the worst kind of fat — trans fat. Certainly avoid using it yourself but you are more likely to be unwittingly consuming it in processed, packaged foods.

STICK/BLOCK MARGARINES	These are more solid margarines used as a cheap alternative to butter. The problem is that oil is liquid at room temperature. Therefore to make a solid product the oil has to be structurally changed to be more similar to saturated fat (think of fluid olive oil compared to hard butter). The result is the significant production of trans fats. We can think of no reason to ever use these products.
SUET AND TALLOW	Suet is raw beef or mutton fat and tallow is made from suet. Both are high in saturated fat. While you may not ever think you consume these fats, they are used in many foods such as pastries. Vegetable suet is made from palm oil and is therefore not much better.
VISIBLE MEAT FAT 	The solid, white fat you can see on meat, under the skin on poultry, in salami and sausages, and marbled through many meats is a major source of unhealthy saturated fat and cholesterol. Remove it where you can and choose lean cuts of meat without marbling.

Note: In our overall diets, we want to ensure we don't allow the polyunsaturated omega-6 fats to dominate over the omega-3s. A balance of the two fat types is crucial. Oils are the pure fat extracted from the nut or seed and are therefore a far more significant source of the fat than eating the whole food. For this reason we don't include omega-6–rich oils in our 5-star choices because a better choice is a neutral monounsaturated fat or oil that provides omega 3s. However, nuts and seeds that contain omega-6s have other nutritional attributes and the total amount of fat you get from eating the whole food is far less, therefore most of these are included as 5-star fats.

DRINKS

Each drink was assigned a rating based on its nutritional profile. The criteria were based on the drink's ability to hydrate the body without negatively influencing its performance. Consideration was given to energy density, antioxidants/phytochemicals, nutrients, added sugars and sweeteners, and other processing factors.

DRINK	Nutrient Summary
FRESH VEGETABLE JUICE ☆ ☆ ☆ ☆ ☆	Low energy density and packed with nutrients. A good way to boost your veggie intake. Juice your own or buy one with no undesirable additives.
HERBAL TEAS ☆ ☆ ☆ ☆ ☆	Most are calorie free. Herbal teas are a caffeine-free alternative to coffee and tea. Some have mild therapeutic benefits, such as chamomile to aid sleep. However, in excess, some can discolor the enamel of your teeth.
ROOIBOS TEA ☆ ☆ ☆ ☆ ☆	Another calorie and caffeine-free drink. Rooibos is a red leaf tea from South Africa. Rich in antioxidants. It can be drunk with or without milk and makes a good caffeine-free alternative to tea.
SPARKLING OR STILL MINERAL WATER ☆ ☆ ☆ ☆ ☆	Calorie free and provides small quantities of minerals. The bubbles can make a refreshing change and can help if you're trying to cut back on soft drinks or reduce alcohol intake at night.
TEA — BLACK, GREEN, WHITE, AND OOLONG ☆ ☆ ☆ ☆ ☆	All these teas are a rich source of antioxidants, and tea drinking is associated with a lower risk of heart disease and several cancers including stomach, esophageal, skin, and ovarian cancer. Green tea is not to everyone's taste and can make some people slightly nauseous. Take heart that, despite this tea's good publicity, all tea promotes good health. Do be aware that all tea, including green, contains caffeine (less than half the amount found in coffee), but the caffeine intake from drinking four to five cups of tea a day is not associated with any harmful effects. Tea also contains tannins that inhibit the absorption of plant-based iron. Avoid this problem by drinking your tea between, and not with, your meals.

DRINK	*Nutrient Summary*
WATER ☆ ☆ ☆ ☆ ☆	Calorie free and quite simply the best and cheapest way to hydrate the body. No distinction is made here between tap, filtered, and bottled water — bottled water is not necessarily better for your health. Tap water can, in some parts of the country, taste unpleasant. If that's the case where you live, buy bottled or invest in a filter.
FRESH VEGETABLE AND FRUIT JUICE ☆ ☆ ☆ ☆	With the added fruit the energy density increases but it is still a nutrient-rich drink and the fruit makes it more palatable than plain vegetable juice for most people. Make sure the ratio of vegetables to fruit is more than 2:1, only using the fruit to make it slightly sweet.
NATURAL COCOA POWDER (NOT TO BE CONFUSED WITH DRINKING-CHOCOLATE POWDER, WHICH HAS FAR LESS COCOA, ADDED SUGAR, AND OFTEN ADDITIONAL FLAVORINGS AND ADDITIVES) ☆ ☆ ☆ ☆	The native Kuna Indians of Panama drink three to four cups of homemade cocoa a day and have very low rates of high blood pressure and heart disease. Researchers have attributed this to the high flavonoid antioxidants in cocoa. Natural cocoa powder is the least-processed form of chocolate and as such it retains far higher levels of these antioxidants. Plus it has no fat and no added sugar. Try adding a teaspoon to warm skim milk for a healthy chocolate fix. However, cocoa does contain small amounts of caffeine and much higher levels of a similar compound called theobromine, which has similar, but far milder, effects on the central nervous system as caffeine does. However, you are extremely unlikely to consume enough cocoa powder for this to be a problem!
SODA WATER ☆ ☆ ☆ ☆	This is just carbonated water, but it is higher in sodium (salt) than most other waters. Nevertheless, it provides calorie-free hydration.

DRINK	*Nutrient Summary*
ALCOHOL, INCLUDING WINE, SPIRITS, AND BEER ☆ ☆ ☆	Wine has had all the good press but, in fact, all alcoholic drinks, when regularly consumed in small amounts, are good for the heart and circulatory system and probably reduce the risk of type 2 diabetes and gallstones. It's true that red wine contains more antioxidants than other drinks and these may be of benefit; but let's be honest, these can be found elsewhere. Don't fool yourself into thinking a bottle of red a night is good for you! In excess, alcohol is incredibly harmful, damaging your liver, your heart, increasing your risk of breast cancer and depression, while clouding your judgment and affecting what you choose to eat. By all means enjoy a couple of drinks a day, but give yourself at least two alcohol-free days a week.
COFFEE ☆ ☆ ☆	There are many potential health benefits from coffee (see pages 94–95). For example, it improves alertness, concentration, brain performance, and exercise performance, and may assist weight control by encouraging fat "burning" and boosting metabolism. It also stimulates bowel movement, a welcome relief for many. Like tea, coffee contains a high level of antioxidants, but unlike tea there is no solid evidence that coffee consumption reduces the risk of heart disease and cancer (but neither is there evidence to suggest coffee increases your risk). Coffee (and caffeine) consumption has been shown to lower the risk of Parkinson's disease and diabetes. However, it has more than double the caffeine content of tea, and in excess this can overly stimulate the central nervous system resulting in restlessness, insomnia, anxiety, and tremors. Some people find that coffee irritates the stomach and may make conditions such as heartburn worse. Drinking more than four cups of coffee a day may increase your risk of osteoporosis. Finally, be discerning about what you put in your coffee — whole milk or cream, sugars, and flavored syrups can result in a calorie-packed drink. Stick to a maximum of three a day, use skim milk if you like, and don't add sugar.

DRINK	Nutrient Summary
DECAFFEINATED COFFEE USING THE SWISS WATER® PROCESS ☆ ☆ ☆	This method uses only water to remove the caffeine and is therefore completely chemical free, unlike most other decaf coffees. For information on where you can buy it visit www.swisswater.com. Of course, the removal of the caffeine may also remove some of the benefits of regular coffee. Note: If you suffer from heartburn, studies have shown no difference between decaf and regular coffee, suggesting that the caffeine is not to blame.
FRESH FRUIT JUICE ☆ ☆ ☆	A nutrient-rich drink that is healthy in small amounts. But many nutrients from the whole fruit are lost, especially fiber. Significant source of extra calories since it is relatively energy-dense, and serving sizes can be enormous making it very easy to overconsume. Better to eat the whole fruit instead. Enjoy the occasional fresh juice when you are out, but don't keep it in the fridge at home.
LOW-FAT FRUIT SMOOTHIES MADE WITH FRUIT, LOW-FAT MILK, AND YOGURT WITH NO ADDITIVES ☆ ☆ ☆	Smoothies can be a healthy, satisfying, and filling snack or meal, provided they are made with the right ingredients. Use low-fat milk and yogurt combined with fresh or frozen fruit. The combination is low GI and can be helpful in keeping you full until the next meal. Good breakfast option for those who don't like solid food first thing in the morning. Be wary of the enormous serving sizes, added cream or ice cream, and various undesirable additives that can be found in commercial smoothies.

SKIM MILK ☆ ☆ ☆	All the calcium and protein of whole milk with none of the fat. The protein in milk is also rich in the amino acid leucine, which is thought to assist in preserving muscle (and therefore increasing fat loss) during weight loss and promoting growth and repair of muscles after exercise. The combination of calcium and leucine may be particularly beneficial during weight loss although this has yet to be substantiated. Also has a low GI and can help keep hunger at bay between meals. A warm cup of milk before bed can help you to fall asleep. However, milk is not suitable for those with lactose intolerance and there is some concern that high intakes may increase the risk of ovarian and prostate cancers. Until this is resolved, we cannot be confident about the safety of a high intake of milk. Stick to one to two cups a day to gain the benefits while limiting any potential risks.
CHEMICALLY DECAFFEINATED COFFEE ☆ ☆	Most decaf coffee is made using beans that have had the caffeine removed using chemical solvents. There is inevitably residue of the chemicals present (albeit in small quantities), but whether this has any effect on health is not known. However, one U.S. study found that decaf, and not regular coffee, increased heart disease risk. The reason is not known and one study is not definitive proof. Nevertheless, it cautions us not to make the assumption that decaf must be healthier.
FLAVORED MILK ☆ ☆	Contains a lot of sugar and/or artificial sweeteners and many contain additional artificial flavorings and other additives. They are also usually bought in large sizes — the label will say it contains two or more servings but who only drinks half the bottle? They are, however, low GI and okay for an occasional filling snack when you are on the run. For a healthier choice, choose one that is made with low-fat milk, advertises a lower sugar content, and read the ingredients list to be sure there are no other additives.

DRINK	*Nutrient Summary*
FLAVORED WATER ☆ ☆	Marketed as healthy, but these are just water with added sugar and flavorings. Certainly they have less sugar and fewer calories than soft drinks, but it is much better to make your own with sparkling water and a splash of fruit juice.
FRUIT AND VEGETABLE JUICES WITH ADDED PRESERVATIVES AND COLOR ☆ ☆	Read the label — many seemingly "fresh" fruit and vegetable juices have undesirable additives.
HOT CHOCOLATE ☆ ☆	Although some good qualities in the cocoa, drinking chocolate has a lot of sugar added and sometimes has artificial flavors, preservatives, and other additives too. Read the label. Hot chocolate in cafés can also be loaded with the addition of cream and/or whole milk. They also tend to use a lot of drinking-chocolate powder. Ask for skim milk and less powder.
WINE COOLERS AND OTHER FLAVORED, ALCOHOLIC DRINKS ☆	Sometimes called "girly" drinks, these are a dreadful combination of too much sugar, alcohol, flavorings, colorings, and other additives. They are too easy to drink quickly and to drink too many of. Have a glass of wine and a second with sparkling water instead.
CORDIAL ☆	Extremely high in sugar and often has added artificial colors, flavors, and preservatives.
DIET SOFT DRINKS ☆	Sorry, we are just not fans. They might be almost calorie free, but they use artificial sweeteners, colors, and flavorings, and they still damage your teeth by eroding the enamel. If you need to lose weight they are a step in the right direction from regular soft drinks, but quickly move on and get into the water-drinking habit instead!

DRINK	Nutrient Summary
ENERGY DRINKS ☆	These might sound like a good idea when you need a lift, but they are just soft drinks with added caffeine — and usually lots of it. Be aware that guarana might be all "natural," but it is just more caffeine. The calorie content is often even higher than in regular soft drinks.
SOFT DRINKS/ SODAS ☆	Full of sugar, soft drinks provide package of calories that is all too easy to overconsume, and because of this they play a major role in our escalating weight problem. They are also incredibly bad for your teeth, promoting both decay and erosion. Just don't drink them.

TREATS

The table below summarizes the attributes of each treat. The criteria for the selection process were based on their ability to provide pleasure without doing too much damage. Consideration was given to the energy density, type of fat, processing factors, and the quantity of sugar and/or salt added.

TREAT	Nutrient Summary
DARK CHOCOLATE (AT LEAST 70 PERCENT COCOA) ☆ ☆ ☆ ☆	The cocoa in chocolate is a rich source of flavonoid antioxidants, which are thought to be beneficial to health. They may be cardioprotective by preventing the damage to LDL-cholesterol that results in atherosclerosis and may also lower blood pressure. Dark chocolate contains the most cocoa and therefore the highest level of antioxidants. There is little difference in fat or calories between dark, milk, and white chocolate, but the strong, slightly bitter flavor of dark chocolate tends to satisfy you and put a brake on how much you eat. Although high in saturated fat, the type found in cocoa butter does not raise cholesterol. (The same may not be true for lower-quality chocolate made with cheaper fats.) This is still an energy-dense food nonetheless, so exercise quality over quantity.
FRUIT BREAD ☆ ☆ ☆ ☆	Dense fruit bread made with whole-wheat flour and lots of fruit has a low GI (which is not the case for many commercial sliced raisin toast varieties). In addition, the dried fruit provides many nutrients (covered in our fruit section). Delicious served with low-fat ricotta. Read the labels of commercial varieties — many have undesirable additives including preservatives — and look for one with a simple list of all food ingredients.

TREAT	*Nutrient Summary*
100 PERCENT FRUIT BARS/ ROLL-UPS ☆ ☆ ☆ ☆	Although they're not a good as fresh fruit, these treats are a handy, no-mess addition to a school lunchbox. With many of the nutrients of fresh fruit, they're easy to transport and provide a great source of energy. Make sure you check the labels before purchase — not all are 100 percent fruit, and some have added sugar, flavors, colors, and other artificial additives. This also affects their GI. While those made with 100 percent fruit are shown to have low GIs, those with 65 percent fruit or less can have extremely high GI values.
WHOLE-WHEAT, FRUIT-FILLED BARS AND COOKIES ☆ ☆ ☆ ☆	A higher-fiber snack than most sweets and lower in refined sugar. Search the GI database for those with a low GI for the best choice (www.glycemicindex.com).
MIXED DRIED FRUIT WITH RAW NUTS AND SEEDS (TRAIL MIX) ☆ ☆ ☆ ☆	A good high-fiber, low-GI snack but far more energy-dense than fresh fruit. Enjoy in moderation. Drying fruit is essentially a great way to preserve fresh fruit and give it a conveniently long shelf life. Most nutrients are preserved with the exception of vitamin C. Sulphur dioxide is usually added to commercial dried fruits to keep their bright color. You can avoid this additive by choosing organic, sun-dried fruit — it will be darker in color but the flavor is usually also better. Adding raw nuts and seeds adds fiber, protein, and healthy fats for a more balanced, filling snack.
ROASTED, UNSALTED NUTS ☆ ☆ ☆ ☆	Roasted nuts may become rancid if they are stored for too long. Provided you buy them from a store with a quick turnover, they make a good snack. They do have a high energy density, so be careful not to overeat. A standard serving is around 30 grams, the equivalent to approximately 30 almonds, 10 brazil nuts, or 20 cashews.
HOMEMADE OAT/ MUESLI BARS ☆ ☆ ☆ ☆	Made with raw muesli and a small amount of butter and sugar, homemade muesli bars make a good high-fiber snack with all the nutrients found in muesli.
AIR-POPPED CORN ☆ ☆ ☆	Cooked with no fat or added sugar, popcorn is a good high-fiber, low-energy snack. It has a high GI, so don't expect it to fill you up. Avoid it if you're managing high blood sugar.

TREAT	*Nutrient Summary*
BISCOTTI ☆ ☆ ☆	Traditional biscotti contain no oil or butter and is therefore a low-fat treat. They are made with white flour and sugar, but the almonds help to reduce their GI and boost their overall nutritional value. Many recipes add chocolate chunks, cocoa powder, etc., and are not as good as plain biscotti.
BANANA BREAD (WITHOUT ICING) ☆ ☆ ☆	Largely dependent on the recipe and the type of flour, fat, and quantity of sugar used, some nutrients from the banana make this treat better than many others.
CARROT CAKE (WITHOUT ICING) ☆ ☆ ☆	Largely dependent on the recipe and the type of flour, fat, and quantity of sugar used, some nutrients from the carrot make this treat better than many others.
BRAN AND FRUIT MUFFINS ☆ ☆ ☆	Another treat that is largely dependent on the recipe (and SIZE!). Select muffins made with part whole-wheat flour, fruit, and bran that are no bigger than 2¾ inches in diameter. They make a reasonable, high-fiber snack.
FRUIT CAKE ☆ ☆ ☆	A dense fruit cake is a high-energy snack, but offers a number of nutrients and fiber from the fruit.
HOMEMADE FRUIT PIES AND CRUMBLES ☆ ☆ ☆	Made from naturally sweet fruit with little added sugar and a pastry or crumble top, these are not too bad.
CHOCOLATE-COVERED NUTS AND RAISINS ☆ ☆ ☆	The health benefits of the nuts and raisins are offset by the low-quality, high-sugar/high-fat chocolate coating.
MILK CHOCOLATE ☆ ☆ ☆	Higher in fat and sugar than dark chocolate but still contains some of the health benefits from the cocoa.
WHEAT/OAT CRACKERS ☆ ☆ ☆	Some fiber from the wheat and oats.
SALTED/TAMARI-ROASTED NUTS ☆ ☆ ☆	A good source of fiber and other nutrients from nuts, but easy to overeat. High in energy and salt.

— *101 Healthiest Foods* —

TREAT	*Nutrient Summary*
REAL LICORICE ☆ ☆ ☆	Licorice comes from the root of a shrub 50 times sweeter than sugar. The candy is made from molasses with small quantities of licorice and anise. Molasses is a thick syrup byproduct produced during the production of table sugar. It contains small amounts of several nutrients including iron, magnesium, vitamin K, and potassium, but it is still primarily extracted sugar, so don't be fooled into thinking it is a health product. When buying licorice, check the ingredients to ensure it's made from molasses; cheaper versions are artificially flavored candy and not the real thing. A serving should be no greater than one 4-inch piece.
COMMERCIAL FRUIT PIES ☆ ☆	Commercially bought pies are often loaded with sugar. With both a top and a bottom crust, they are high in energy and some are made with damaging trans fats.
MUFFINS ☆ ☆	Made from white, processed flour and sugar and are generally oversized. High GI.
BOXED CHOCOLATES ☆ ☆	Candy and toffee fillings are full of sugar and many other commercial additives.
CARAMELIZED NUTS ☆ ☆	Very high in refined sugar and not great for your teeth.
SCONES ☆ ☆	High GI, made with white, bleached flour and fat.
WHITE CHOCOLATE ☆ ☆	Made from fat and sugar with no cocoa.
CHOCOLATE-COVERED COOKIES ☆ ☆	Poor-quality chocolate, high fat and sugar contents, and added colorings make these a poor choice.
GRANOLA BARS ☆ ☆	Generally thought of as healthy, they are very high in sugar (from glucose) and high in fat. A very high-calorie food.

TREAT	*Nutrient Summary*
PANCAKES ☆ ☆	High GI, made with white, bleached flour and fat. Premixed commercial pancake products have extra additives and are even worse.
SPONGE CAKES AND CUPCAKES (WITHOUT ICING) ☆ ☆	High GI, bleached, white flour, butter, and sugar form the basis of all sponge cakes.
PRETZELS ☆ ☆	Marketed as a healthy snack, they have an exceptionally high GI and are high in salt.
SOY CHIPS ☆ ☆	Considered healthy, soy chips are deep-fried and high in salt and energy.
SALTED CHIPS ☆ ☆	High in salt and energy — like all salted products, easy to overeat.
HOMEMADE OR QUALITY ICE CREAM ☆ ☆	Made from thickened cream and sugar, which are natural ingredients and therefore a far better choice than those loaded with artificial additives and flavors. However, high in saturated fat and high-calorie, so not an everyday food.
HARD CANDY ☆	Made from boiled sugar, water, and artificial coloring and flavors. At best they work on rotting the teeth.
JELLY AND JELLIED CANDY ☆	Sugar, artificial coloring, and additives.
ICED SPONGE CAKES, CUPCAKES, AND CREAM CAKES ☆	High GI, bleached, white flour, butter, and sugar form the basis of all sponges. Cream and icing lift the fat and sugar content making them worse, and adding coloring to the icing worse again.
CHOCOLATE CAKES AND BROWNIES ☆	Loaded in fat and sugar, these are very high in calories.

TREAT	Nutrient Summary
CHOCOLATE-COVERED TOFFEE ☆	Very high in calories and refined sugar. The stickiness makes these treats a disaster for teeth.
COMMERCIAL ICE CREAM, INCLUDING NOVELTIES ☆	Made from poor-quality vegetable fat and sugar, usually with added artificial flavorings and coloring. Lots of calories for very few nutrients.
CHEESECAKE ☆	High in saturated fat and calories.
NOUGAT ☆	Boiled sugar, with coloring and a few nuts.
CORN DOGS ☆	Deep-fried, battered hot dogs — high in saturated fat and loaded with calories. Also likely to contain trans fats.
PROTEIN BARS ☆	Marketed as healthy, but why should processed protein be any better for us than processed anything else? In addition they are often full of artificial additives and flavorings.
FLAVORED CHIPS AND SNACK MIXES ☆	High concentration of salt and artificial flavorings. Energy dense and full of the wrong types of fat.
SWEET PASTRIES ☆	High GI, loaded with calories and the wrong types of fat.
CREAMY DESSERTS ☆	Energy-dense and high in saturated fat, cholesterol, and sugar.
DOUGHNUTS ☆	Deep-fried, white, processed flour and lots of sugar. Glazed doughnuts are even worse.
PANCAKE AND CAKE MIXES ☆	Have extra additives to preserve the main ingredients.

Part 3: Recipes

COOKING AND RECIPES

If you think of cooking as a chore, it will always be one. If you see it as a creative expression, you may see yourself as an artist. It's a better option than feeling like a slave to the kitchen and a servant to those you cook for. Best of all, what you cook will taste much better.

I didn't train as a chef or learn how to cook at school. I write this to anyone who has reached this section of the book and is now saying it's too hard to cook and you simply don't have the time to do it. I learned to cook because I like eating and I like eating good food. Being vain and having a tendency to gain fat, I started with the desire to eat the types of food that helped maintain my body size. And I felt better for it.

Now in my 40s, I want to stay fit, active, and as young looking as possible. Were I in my 50s I might be saying I wanted to avoid chronic disease, and in my 60s I'll probably be saying I want to reach a ripe old age. Whatever your motivation is, the fact is you'll feel better at any age if you make a choice to get into the kitchen and learn how to prepare easy, healthy meals using fresh, natural ingredients.

Suspend disbelief about your ability in the kitchen and recognize that anyone can learn anything with a little invested time and practice. With that in mind, it's handy to know that most modern recipes, including the majority in this chapter, can be made in around 30 minutes — less time than it would take for take-out to be delivered!

The tricks of a healthy eater

If you've been a 1- or 2-star eater most of your days, you have a bit of work to do, but, like anything new, what starts off feeling difficult and uncomfortable will in time become surprisingly simple.

Here are the tricks of the healthy eater.

OUT WITH THE OLD
With your food hierarchies as a guide, go through your refrigerator and freezer and throw out all the 1- and 2-star foods. And if you order take-out most nights of the week, throw the menus out as well.

THE BASIC TOOLS TO MAKE COOKING EASIER

You don't have to buy an entire kitchen collection, but there are some basics you do need to get food on the table quickly and efficiently, and they don't need to cost you a fortune.

Check the list of kitchen items below and stock up with the things you don't have:

ITEM	WHY YOU NEED IT
2 baking trays	To roast veggies, etc.
1 baking sheet	To finish off meat and fish.
1 griddle pan	To sear or grill meat, fish, and veggies.
2 cutting boards	One for veggies and fruit, the other for meat and fish.
Sieve or colander	For draining grains and veggies.
Food processor	The quickest way to make sauces and pastry and blend soups.
Heavy oven-proof frying pan with lid	For stove-top and oven cooking, to sauté and make hearty casseroles.
Garlic press	A great time saver.
Jar with lid	Any jar will do to make and mix salad dressings in.
Multisize grater	Large holes for cheese and veggies, smaller holes for ginger, Parmesan cheese, and nutmeg.
Knives	No compromise here — a couple of good quality knives make an enormous difference in the kitchen. Ideally you want a large heavy multipurpose blade, a smaller knife to use on small items, and a small serrated blade for trimming around veggies and fruit peels.
Ladle	Useful for soups and soupy casseroles.
Measuring spoons and cups	There's less need to measure most 5-star foods, but in some recipes if you don't they'll either not taste so great or won't work. Besides, a careless extra slurp of olive oil amounts to an additional 160 unnecessary calories, which is less than useful when you want to lose weight.
Mixing bowls	A set of stainless steel bowls are everyday musts; used to mix grains for breakfast cereal, toss salad leaves, beat eggs, etc.

Salad spinner	This will sway those who skip the salad on the side because they can't be bothered to wash and dry the greens. With salad greens washed and dried in seconds and a dressing whipped up in a couple of minutes, a side salad will become part of everyday eating.
Scissors	Handy to open sealed plastic packaging.
Large slotted spoon	To remove poached eggs, also very handy when serving thick, chunky veggie soup.
Small pancake or omelet pan	Handy for dry roasting nuts and seeds, and (obviously) making omelets and pancakes!
Spatula	Essential.
Stainless steel saucepans	Buy quality pans — a large stockpot for pasta and soups, a medium pan, and a small pan are a good basic starting kit.
Steamer	Buy a stainless steel steamer to fit on one of your pans. A bamboo steamer is a cheaper alternative.
Tongs	Forget the long tongs which give you no control whatsoever; a small pair to turn meat and fish and serve with is essential.
Vegetable peeler	For the obvious and to grate cheese.
Wok	If your stove is electric, buy an electric wok. If you have a gas stove, a large cast-iron wok makes an easy and delicious stir-fry in minutes.
Wooden spoons	A couple are useful.

Shopping

There are a number of online websites you can use these days to make shopping easier and faster, but most people still prefer to get out to the stores and select their own fresh produce. It entirely depends on what you can make time for. Ideally, you'll be able to make time for a big trip (usually on the weekend) and a mini trip later in the week to pick up a few extra perishables for the remainder of the week. Fresh fish is best eaten on the day it's bought or, at the latest, the day after. Meat, provided it's well wrapped, will be fine refrigerated for up to 4 days. If you buy it vacuum packed it lasts even longer. Leafy vegetables, stored in plastic bags in the refrigerator, will be good for up to 4 days. Root vegetables and harder vegetables such as sweet potato, onion, carrot, and garlic will store in the pantry for a couple of weeks. Here are some more tips:

- Depending on the number of people you're cooking for, you should be able to stock up your healthy pantry and fridge with one big shopping trip and one smaller trip later in the week.

- On the big shopping trip you'll buy the labor-saving foods and the perishables. Labor-saving foods are things like canned tomatoes, canned legumes, canned fish, natural preservative stocks, pasta sauces, condiments such as tamari, tahini, reduced-sodium soy sauce, preserved lemons, oils, vinegar, tea, bottled water, nuts and seeds, mixed grains, dried fruit, herbs and spices, frozen berries, and frozen veggies. The perishables include fresh meat, fresh fish, low-fat dairy, and as many fruits and vegetables to get you by until the next smaller shopping trip.

- The small trip is to refill enough of the perishable foods to see you through to the end of the week. Depending on where you live, it may be more enjoyable to do the mini shop at the local shops with a green grocer, butcher, and (hopefully) a fish shop and save the large shop for the major shopping center.

WHEN TO SHOP

If you work Monday to Friday, it may seem like a drag allocating a couple of hours to grocery shopping on one of your valuable days off, but, if you do it when you have time to spare, you're more likely to plan properly and less likely to forget anything. You'll also have time to unpack and store your produce properly when you get home. If you get off to an early start, you'll hit the stores before the crowds and have the rest of the day to eat well and have fun.

Don't panic — you won't have to go grocery shopping every Saturday or Sunday for the rest of your life. In time the process will become easier, and you'll master it sufficiently to whip around the store in half the time.

Farmers markets, fish markets, and food purveyors make buying fresh produce a great day out so it's well worth investigating what's going on in your area.

BREAKFASTS

Some people say breakfast is their favorite meal of the day. Observing them, they're generally slim, full of energy, glowing with health, and positive. Others say they don't feel like eating first thing in the morning. Observing them, they're often none of the things described above.

Research backs up these observations, particularly in relation to weight control — breakfast eaters really are slimmer. Whether you have to eat less or earlier at night, or get up earlier to exercise so you build an appetite, it's worth doing. Breakfast is the meal that breaks the fast from the long night's sleep. It boosts your metabolism, gives you the energy to get through the morning's activities, and helps you maintain focus and attention.

TRIPLE GRAIN MUESLI

Serves 20

It's unlikely you'll ever find prunes in commercial muesli because they tend to clump together if they're chopped in an electric processor. You'll have to chop them by hand and add them to the grains a few at a time. It's also worth grinding your own ground flaxseeds, sunflower seeds, and almonds rather than buying them ground from a health food store. It's fresher and the texture is less like sand. Grind them just long enough to break up the seeds but keep the almonds crunchy. It might seem like a chore to make your own muesli, but it really is worth the effort. At the end of the day, you've made a delicious, premium muesli in which every single ingredient rates as a 5-star food.

1 cup raw almonds

1 cup sunflower seeds

1 cup flaxseeds

2 cups rolled oats

2 cups rolled barley flakes

2 cups rolled rye flakes

½ cup dried apricots, roughly chopped

1 cup pitted prunes, roughly chopped

METHOD

1. Grind the almonds, sunflower seeds, and flaxseeds in a food processor.

2. Combine with the rolled grains. Add the dried fruit slowly and stir as you go to prevent the fruit clumping together.

3. Store in the refrigerator in an airtight container.

4. Serve with fresh fruit, low-fat natural yogurt, and flaxseed oil.

BUCKWHEAT PANCAKES WITH BLUEBERRY SAUCE AND HONEY YOGURT

Serves 6

Here's a nice breakfast for the whole family to enjoy. Even though berries are not in season during winter, you can always use frozen — nutritionally they're just as good and they're much cheaper.

2 pints blueberries

4 tablespoons honey

1 tablespoon lemon juice

¾ cup buckwheat flour

¼ cup whole-wheat flour, sifted

sea salt

2 free-range eggs

1½ cups buttermilk

½ cup water

1½ cups low-fat plain yogurt

olive or grapeseed oil

1 pint strawberries, to serve

1 pint raspberries, to serve

METHOD

1. In a small pan, slowly bring a pint of blueberries to the boil with 1 tablespoon water, 2 tablespoons honey, and the lemon juice. Cover and reduce the heat to a slow simmer for 3 minutes until the berries have stewed.

2. Mix in a blender until very smooth.

3. Sift the flours and a pinch of sea salt into a bowl. Make a well in the center and add the eggs. Beat the eggs into the flour.

4. Gradually add the buttermilk and water and beat until bubbles form on the surface of the pancake batter. Cover and refrigerate until ready to use.

5. Add the remaining honey to the yogurt, beat together, and refrigerate.

6. Using a paper towel and olive or grapeseed oil, lightly oil a small pancake pan.

7. Beat the pancake mixture once again before transferring into a jug for easy pouring.

8. Pour enough batter into the pan to cover the bottom and make a pancake approximately 4 mm thick.

9. Cook for 3–4 minutes or until bubbles form on the surface of the pancake.

10. Flip the pancake and cook for another minute.

11. Repeat the process until the batter mix is finished.

12. Top with honey yogurt and blueberry sauce and serve with berries.

A SLIGHT BREAK
FROM TRADITION — OATMEAL

Serves 4

Traditional Scottish porridge is made with steel-cut oats, water and salt, although no one I know likes it like that (except Joanna's mom!). Nowadays porridge is made using a variety of oats including rolled oats, quick oats, and instant oats. The less processed the oats are, the lower the GI of the oatmeal is. Therefore, while it may take longer to cook, oatmeal made from steel-cut oats is the healthiest choice. By breaking from tradition with added ginger, fruit, and nuts, we create a far more interesting and delicious meal with numerous health attributes in addition to those from oats alone. This dish can be made in the slow cooker and cooked overnight.

1 cup steel-cut oats

6 cups water

1 tablespoon grated fresh ginger

1 green apple cut into rough chunks

1 teaspoon sea salt

1 cup low-fat milk

2 tablespoons walnuts

1 tablespoon pepitas (pumpkin seeds)

6 dried apricots, finely chopped

METHOD

1. Soak the oats in water overnight.

2. Drain thoroughly and place the oats in a pan with the water, ginger, apple, and sea salt.

3. Bring to the boil and then reduce the heat to simmer for 50 minutes, stirring occasionally until most of the water has absorbed and the grain is soft.

4. Add the low-fat milk, nuts, seeds, and apricots and stir through.

Tip: *Delicious served with fresh fruit and a tablespoon of honey and soy or low-fat milk or yogurt.*

STRAWBERRY BREAKFAST TRIFLE

Serves 4

Here's an excellent start to the day — if you don't have a sweet tooth you can omit the maple syrup, particularly if the strawberries are sweet. Children may find it more approachable with the syrup added and, if it helps them eat oats and seeds, it's well worth adding.

2 cups rolled oats

2 tablespoons almonds

2 tablespoons sunflower seeds

2 tablespoons pepitas (pumpkin seeds)

2 tablespoons maple syrup

1 large container of strawberries, washed, hulled, and cut into quarters

8 ounces low-fat natural yogurt

METHOD

1. Preheat oven to 350°F.

2. Coat the oats, nuts, and seeds with maple syrup and lay out on a flat baking sheet lined with parchment paper.

3. Place in the middle of the oven and dry-roast for approximately 8 minutes, turning the mixture regularly with a spoon to prevent it from burning.

4. Remove from the oven and set aside.

5. In a glass dish, arrange a layer of strawberries on the bottom, then a layer of the oat and seed mixture, and top with natural yogurt; repeat the process, finishing with a few strawberries for garnish.

BREAKFAST QUINOA

Serves 4–6

Many commercial, gluten-free breakfast cereals have a high GI. This breakfast quinoa is suitable for people who can't eat wheat and/or gluten, and it also has a low GI to sustain energy throughout the morning. Apple juice concentrate is a natural sweetener available from health food stores. This will store for up to 3 days in the refrigerator.

2 cups quinoa

2½ cups cold water

1 cinnamon stick

½ cup apple juice concentrate

½ cup mixed chopped nuts (almonds, Brazil nuts, walnuts)

¼ cup dried apricots, chopped

fresh fruit or stewed fruit compote, to serve

low-fat natural yogurt, to serve

METHOD

1. Thoroughly rinse and drain the quinoa.

2. Add the quinoa to a pan with the water, cinnamon stick, and apple concentrate and bring to a boil. Reduce to a simmer and cover.

3. Cook for 15 minutes until the quinoa is tender and the liquid has absorbed into the grain.

4. While the quinoa is cooking, dry-roast the nuts in a frying pan until they're golden and fragrant.

5. Stir the nuts and chopped apricots through the quinoa and serve with fresh or stewed fruit and yogurt.

ENTRÉES AND LIGHT MEALS

Even if you're not that hungry at mealtimes, you should still make the effort to make a light meal incorporating a few 5-star ingredients. It's another opportunity to feed your body the nutrients it needs to power through the day. Compared to eating one or two large meals, eating more frequent smaller meals helps you to manage your weight better and gives your body a chance to absorb all those wonderful nutrients throughout the course of the day rather than being bombarded with an enormous load all at once. The latter is likely to leave you lethargic, bloated, and, if it is late at night, unable to sleep well.

SPICY ROASTED NUTS

Serves 4–6

These nuts make a nice snack to serve with before-dinner drinks. They're much healthier than commercial varieties and, when served warm, they are much more delicious.

1 cup mixed raw nuts (including cashews, almonds, walnuts, and Brazil nuts)

½ tablespoon olive oil

½ teaspoon fine sea salt

pinch chili flakes

METHOD

1 Preheat the oven to 400°F.

2 Line a baking tray with parchment paper.

3 Lay the nuts on the sheet and sprinkle the olive oil over them, shaking them gently on the tray to ensure each nut is lightly coated with oil.

4 Sprinkle sea salt and chili flakes over them and stir through.

5 Place the tray in the oven and roast for 4–5 minutes. Stir to allow the nuts to roast evenly and roast for a further 4 minutes.

Note: *Nuts can turn rancid or moldy if they've been stored too long or left unsealed in a warm place. To avoid rancidity, and the risk of free-radical damage from eating rancid nuts, buy raw nuts and store them in a sealed jar in the refrigerator.*

AVOCADO GAZPACHO

Serves 6

Packed with 5-star ingredients, this cold soup can also be used as a dressing over salad greens and fresh prawns. Store in the refrigerator for up to five days in an airtight container.

3 small, ripe avocados

1 Persian cucumber, roughly chopped

1 green bell pepper, seeded

1 green chili, seeded

1 red onion, peeled

2 cloves garlic, peeled

2 cups cold, filtered water

1 teaspoon sea salt

1 bunch cilantro

juice of 1 lime

cracked black pepper

To serve

½ cup low-fat plain yogurt

pinch smoked paprika

limes, quartered

METHOD

1. Skin, halve, and pit avocados.

2. Using a juicer, juice the cucumber, bell pepper, chili, onion, and garlic.

3. Combine the vegetable juice, avocados, water, salt, cilantro, lime juice, and black pepper in a blender and process thoroughly.

4. Serve chilled, with a dollop of low-fat plain yogurt, a
   sprinkle of smoked paprika, lime quarters, and cracked
   pepper.

Tip: *If you don't use a whole avocado right away, replace the seed, sprinkle the exposed flesh with lemon juice, and wrap it tightly in foil before refrigerating. Eat within 1 to 2 days of cutting.*

SHIITAKE AND BUCKWHEAT SOUP

Serves 6

This rich-tasting soup is an excellent winter warmer. In Eastern medicine, shiitake mushrooms are reputed to have immune-boosting qualities — another bonus during the season in which we're most prone to bacterial and viral attack.

8 shiitake mushrooms

2 cups hot water

6 cups water

¼ cup buckwheat

2 whole shallots

⅓ inch x 1 inch piece fresh ginger, peeled

2 star anise

3 tablespoons mirin

3 tablespoons tamari

1 carrot, julienned

4 shallots, finely chopped, extra

½ bunch cilantro, chopped

METHOD

1. Place shiitake mushrooms in a bowl and cover with 2 cups hot water. Allow to stand for 20 minutes.

2. Add the soaking water to a saucepan with 6 cups water, buckwheat, whole shallots, ginger, star anise, mirin, and tamari.

3. Bring to a boil slowly and simmer for 20 minutes.

4. Add the carrots and sliced shiitake (stems removed) and cook for another 15 minutes.

5. Remove ginger, shallots, and star anise.

6. Place into serving bowls and add 1 teaspoon each chopped cilantro and chopped shallots.

VEGETARIAN SAN CHOY BAU

Serves 4–6

I challenge people who say they don't like tofu. It's a bit like art and music — you're bound to like some version of it. Most people object to the texture and the fact that tofu doesn't taste like anything. However, this can work to your advantage because tofu will take on the flavors you wish it to in the dish. This recipe does just that and disguises tofu's texture so much that some people could even be fooled into thinking they were eating meat.

12 ounces firm tofu

2 tablespoons pine nuts

1 tablespoon olive oil

10½ ounces mushrooms, finely chopped

1 red chili, finely chopped

3 cilantro roots, scrubbed and crushed

2 tablespoons reduced-sodium soy sauce

4 shallots, thinly sliced

juice of ½ lemon

¼ bunch cilantro leaves

½ savoy cabbage

METHOD

1. Cut the tofu into cubes and place in a pan filled with water.

2. Bring the water to the boil, reduce the heat slightly, and cook until the tofu rises to the surface of the water.

3. Drain the water, blot the tofu dry, and place in a food processor.

4. Mince the tofu into small pieces.

5. In a small pan, dry-roast the pine nuts until golden taking care not to burn them. Remove from the heat and set aside.

6. Heat a wok over a high heat until hot before adding the oil, mushrooms, chili, and crushed cilantro root. Stir-fry for 4 minutes.

7. Add the minced tofu and stir-fry for another 2 minutes. Add the soy sauce and most of the shallots (reserving some for garnish).

8. Stir in the lemon juice, pine nuts, and cilantro leaves.

9. Carefully separate the cabbage leaves and try to keep them whole. Steam the leaves in a bamboo steamer for 5 minutes.

10. Fill each cabbage leaf with the tofu mixture. Top with chopped shallots and, if desired, extra soy sauce for seasoning.

SARDINE, AVOCADO, AND BELL PEPPER GRILL

Serves 4

Here's an easy and substantial meal that tastes great and is packed with nutritional goodies.

12 sardine fillets

olive oil

juice of ½ lemon

4 slices whole-grain bread, toasted

1 avocado

2 tablespoons capers

black pepper

1 cup arugula leaves

1 roasted bell pepper, sliced

METHOD

1. Brush the sardines with olive oil and a sprinkle of lemon juice.

2. Heat a grill pan and cook sardines for 3–4 minutes on one side only.

3. Spread each slice of toast with avocado and sprinkle the capers over the top. Season with black pepper and a little more lemon juice.

4. Lay the arugula over the avocado.

5. Top with sardines and sliced bell pepper and serve.

OYSTERS WITH DICED VEGETABLES AND HERB VINAIGRETTE

Serves 4

Fresh oysters with a squeeze of lemon juice and black pepper are delicious, but, to boost the nutritional value a little more, try chopping a few veggies and herbs over them too.

1 small carrot

1 stick celery

¼ red bell pepper

¼ green bell pepper

1 tablespoon chopped basil

1 tablespoon chopped chervil

3 tablespoons extra-virgin, cold-pressed olive oil

1 tablespoon lemon juice

24 oysters

cracked black pepper

METHOD

1. Finely dice the carrot, celery, and bell peppers. Place in a bowl with the chopped herbs.

2. Stir in the olive oil and lemon juice.

3. Add a spoonful of the vegetable mixture on each oyster.

4. Season with cracked black pepper.

CUCUMBER, EGGPLANT, AVOCADO, AND BULGUR TIMBALE

Serves 4

This impressive-looking dish is a fabulous entrée at any dinner party. It's delicious served on its own with the dressing recipe as shown or with the Avocado Gazpacho (recipe page 169). If you don't have a metal ring, don't worry — on its own as a salad it's still great.

½ cup coarse bulgur

1 cup boiling water

1 small eggplant, finely diced

juice of 1 lemon

2 Persian cucumbers

½ cup chopped parsley

4 vine-ripened tomatoes, peeled, seeded, and chopped

1 avocado, diced

2 tablespoons olive oil

2 teaspoons white balsamic vinegar

1 teaspoon Dijon mustard

1 large clove garlic

METHOD

1. Rinse the bulgur thoroughly then leave it to soak in a bowl with 1 cup boiling water.

2. Finely dice the eggplant and sprinkle the lemon juice over it. Cover and set aside.

3. Drain any excess moisture from the bulgur and combine it with the cucumber, parsley, and tomato.

4. Lay a large metal ring on a plate and fill it with one-quarter of the bulgur and vegetable mix. Top with chopped avocado.

5. Remove the ring and repeat until you have completed 4.

6. Combine the olive oil, vinegar, mustard, and garlic and drizzle a spoonful over each timbale.

LENTIL & FREEKEH PATTIES
WITH COLESLAW

Serves 4

The vegetarians and vegans out there will have to fight their meat-eating friends for a share of these lentil patties. They're a great source of protein and fiber, boosted by combining the grain freekeh with the lentils, and they have a low GI.

Patties

½ cup whole freekeh

1 cup brown lentils

3 cups water

1 tablespoon olive oil

1 small brown onion, peeled, and finely chopped

2 cloves garlic

2 teaspoons cumin

2 teaspoons ground coriander powder

2 pieces preserved lemon or lime, pulp removed, and skin finely chopped

⅓ cup chopped cilantro

sea salt and ground black pepper for seasoning

Coleslaw

1 carrot, grated

2 shallots, sliced

2 cups finely sliced green cabbage

1 cup finely sliced red cabbage

1 cup grated red radish

1 cup sheep's milk yogurt

2 tablespoons lime juice

1 teaspoon maple syrup

1 avocado

cut limes, to serve

METHOD

1. Cook the freekeh according to the instructions on the packet.

2. While the grain is cooking, in a separate pan add the lentils, 3 cups water, and bring to a boil. Reduce the heat and simmer for approximately 30 minutes until the lentils are tender.

3. Drain the freekeh and lentils of any excess water.

4. Place the freekeh and lentils in a food processor and process until they are well combined but retain their texture.

5. Heat the olive oil in a small pan.

6. Add the onions and garlic and sauté for a couple of minutes until tender.

7. Add the spices and cook for another 2 minutes.

8. Transfer the onion mixture to a bowl with the lentils and freekeh.

9. Combine thoroughly with preserved lemon, fresh cilantro, and seasoning.

10. Mold the mixture into flat patties (approx. 3 in × 1 in).

11. Heat a non-stick pan with one tablespoon of olive oil and pan-fry the patties for 3–4 minutes each side.

12. To make the coleslaw, combine the vegetables in a bowl.

13. Mix the yogurt, lime juice, and maple syrup in a separate bowl to make a dressing and combine thoroughly with the coleslaw.

14. Serve over the patties with accompanying slices of fresh avocado and lime juice.

SALADS

We've come a long way from shredded iceberg lettuce, tomato quarters, and a few thick slices of cucumber. Be adventurous with the salad leaves you use; all have different nutrients, tastes, and textures to offer us. Mesclun, the name given to a mix of salad greens, is usually available in most grocery stores and is a good way of including a range of greens without buying each kind individually. Arugula, baby spinach, endive, and watercress are just a few of the many greens available.

A salad can be a meal in itself or a side dish to a main meal. The secret to green salad is choosing a variety of fresh green leaves and serving them in a beautiful shallow bowl. It doesn't have to resemble a supreme pizza with 101 ingredients added. Less is often best.

ASIAN SALAD

Serves 4

4 cups mixed greens

⅓ cup extra-virgin camellia tea oil

1 tablespoon mirin

1 tablespoon brown rice vinegar

½ tablespoon tamari

1 clove garlic, peeled

METHOD

1. Wash and dry the salad greens and place in a mixing bowl.

2. Combine the oil, mirin, brown rice vinegar, and tamari in a small jar.

3. Gently press the flat edge of a knife on the garlic clove to slightly bruise it before dropping it into the jar.

4. Seal and shake the jar to combine the ingredients and set aside for about 30 minutes.

5. Discard the garlic.

6. Shake the jar again and toss the dressing over the leaves.

Note: *1 cup salad greens is the equivalent of 1 serving. If you're at the grocery store buying greens from the salad bin, estimate two tong scoops per person.*

QUINOA TABBOULEH

Serves 6

Bulgur is typically used to make tabbouleh and is another of our 4-star grains. For those who suffer a wheat/gluten intolerance or allergy, this version using quinoa is a terrific alternative.

2 cups quinoa, cooked and cooled (see instruction below)

2 cups parsley, chopped

¼ bunch mint, roughly chopped

¼ bunch arugula, roughly chopped

3 vine-ripened tomatoes, seeded and chopped

juice of 1 lemon

¼ cup extra-virgin olive oil

3 cloves garlic, crushed

1 teaspoon sumac

cracked black pepper

METHOD

1. Cook the quinoa (1 cup quinoa to 2 cups water; bring to a boil; reduce the heat and cover; simmer for 10–15 minutes).

2. Set cooked quinoa aside on a flat dish, spreading it out to allow it to cool evenly.

3. When quinoa is cool, combine all ingredients and serve.

FATOUSH

Serves 4

Fatoush is a Middle Eastern dish traditionally made with pita bread. The bread has been substituted here with sesame seeds. The sesame loads the dish up with more good fats and, in my opinion, makes it much tastier.

Serve as a companion to lamb or chicken with a spoonful of hummus.

1 tablespoon sesame seeds

1 large bunch flat-leaf parsley, roughly chopped

½ bunch mint, roughly chopped

1 bunch baby arugula, roughly chopped

6 shallots, finely sliced

3 vine-ripened tomatoes, roughly chopped

2 Persian cucumbers, finely chopped

3 tablespoons capers, drained and rinsed

juice of 1 lemon

2 cloves garlic, crushed

3 tablespoons extra-virgin olive oil

1 tablespoon sumac

METHOD

1. Dry-roast the sesame seeds in a pan over medium heat until they turn slightly golden. Set aside to cool.

2. Place the prepared greens in a bowl with the shallots, tomato, and cucumber.

3. Chop the capers finely and add them to the bowl.

4. Combine the lemon juice, garlic, olive oil, and sumac in a small bowl, pour it over the salad, and toss until the ingredients are well combined.

Note: *Sumac is a spice that comes from the ripe berries of a Middle Eastern tree. The berries are harvested, partly dried, then ground to remove the purple-red, tangy flesh from the inner seed. The flavor is tangy, lemon-like, salty, and pleasantly acidic. Available from speciality spice stores.*

AVOCADO, MANGO, AND
PINE NUT SALAD

Serves 4

This is perfect for a dinner party. It can be made in minutes just before you and your guests sit down to eat. Dry-roast the pine nuts and make the dressing in advance.

4 tablespoons pine nuts

3 tablespoons extra-virgin, cold-pressed olive oil

1 tablespoon white balsamic vinegar

½ teaspoon Dijon mustard

2 avocados, peeled and sliced

2 mangoes, peeled and sliced

black pepper, to season

— 101 Healthiest Foods —

GREEN SALAD WITH AVOCADO, ALMOND, AND MUSTARD DRESSING

Serves 4

While it's true that with so many good fats this salad is higher in calories than many others, it's so good for you that it's better to cut calories in other ways or increase your exercise than go without these fats.

4 cups mixed greens

½ cup chopped flat-leaf parsley

¼ cup slivered almonds

3 tablespoons extra-virgin olive oil

1 tablespoon white wine vinegar

1 teaspoon whole-grain mustard

cracked black pepper

pinch sea salt

1 large avocado, sliced

METHOD

1. Wash and dry the salad greens and parsley and place them in a mixing bowl.

2. In a small pan, dry-roast the slivered almonds over a medium heat until they turn golden and became fragrant.

3. Combine the oil, vinegar, mustard, and seasoning in a small jar.

4. Pour all but 1 teaspoon of the dressing over the leaves.

5. Toss the leaves and arrange them in a serving dish.

6. Arrange the avocado over the leaves, sprinkle the remaining dressing on, and top with the almond slivers.

Note: *It often happens that a beautiful salad is spoiled after the dressing is tossed in. All the small bits drop to the bottom of the bowl, and if you try to retrieve them, the leaves get knocked around and bruised. The trick to keeping the salad beautiful is to toss the greens with most of the dressing in a large bowl other than the one you're planning to serve the salad in. Once dressed, place them in the serving bowl and top with the other salad items. Then, with a teaspoon, drizzle the remaining dressing over the undressed ingredients.*

GRILLED GOAT CHEESE, HAZELNUT, AND CRANBERRY SALAD

Serves 4

This dish makes a light lunch or entrée.

4 slices whole-grain sourdough bread

7 ounces soft goat cheese

4 teaspoons extra-virgin olive oil

large bunch mixed green salad leaves, washed and dried

½ cup roasted hazelnuts

½ cup cranberry sauce

cracked black pepper

METHOD

1. Toast the bread on one side only under a grill.

2. Remove the bread and lay a couple of pieces of goat cheese on the untoasted side of each slice.

3. Drizzle each slice with a teaspoon of olive oil and return to the grill for another 2–3 minutes.

4. Arrange the salad greens on individual plates and top with the hazelnuts.

5. Lay the toast and goat cheese on the bed of greens, and serve each with a teaspoonful of cranberry sauce and a sprinkling of cracked pepper.

GRILLED SESAME OCTOPUS AND WATERCRESS SALAD

Serves 4

If you don't eat much red meat, it's good to remember that octopus is a great source of iron.

2 tablespoons sesame oil

1 tablespoon lime juice

1 small, red chili pepper, finely chopped

2½ pounds baby octopus, washed and trimmed into small pieces

bunch watercress, washed and trimmed

5 ounces cherry tomatoes, washed

Sesame Dressing

1 tablespoon sesame oil

1 tablespoon olive oil

1 tablespoon lime juice

1 teaspoon soy sauce

1 teaspoon sesame seeds

METHOD

1. Combine the sesame oil, lime juice, and chili and pour over the octopus.

2. Set aside to marinate for 1 hour.

3. Drain the octopus from the marinade.

4. Heat a grill pan to hot and grill the octopus for 3–5 minutes until cooked through.

5. Combine the dressing ingredients in a small jar.

6. Arrange the watercress and tomato on individual plates with the grilled octopus on top.

7. Drizzle with dressing and serve.

SALMON AND CANNELLINI BEAN SALAD

Serves 2

Here's a very easy and healthy lunch to whip up for yourself at home. Make sure you include the bones from the salmon — next to dairy they're the best source of calcium and the crunch factor only adds to the overall dish.

2 cups mixed green salad leaves

1 Persian cucumber, sliced

1 carrot, cut into julienne strips

1½ tablespoons extra-virgin camellia tea oil

1 tablespoon rice vinegar

½ teaspoon grainy mustard

7 ounces canned cannellini beans

1 6½-ounce can red salmon, drained, with the bones remaining

2 small tomatoes, cut into quarters

cracked black pepper

METHOD

1. Wash and dry the salad greens. Combine greens with cucumber and carrot.

2. Combine the camellia tea oil, rice vinegar, and mustard and toss half of the dressing over the leaves, cucumber, and carrots.

3. Drain the cannellini beans and toss the remaining dressing with the beans.

4. Arrange the salad on individual plates.

5. Top with cannellini beans, salmon, and tomatoes and season with black pepper.

Note: *Leftover cannellini beans are delicious puréed with olive oil, garlic, and a little vinegar. Serve as a low-GI dip or as an alternative to mashed potatoes or rice.*

CHICKEN AND POMEGRANATE SALAD

Serves 4

The pomegranate gives this chicken salad a fresh, sweet, tangy taste.

4 organic chicken breasts

1 tablespoon olive oil

3½ ounces raspberries

⅓ cup red wine vinegar

2 tablespoons apple juice concentrate

1 butter-leaf lettuce, washed and dried

1 large avocado, peeled and sliced

1 fennel bulb, thinly sliced

2 stalks celery, finely sliced

7 ounces snow pea sprouts

½ pomegranate, seeded (cut in half with seeds scooped out)

METHOD

1. Preheat the oven to 350°F.

2. Brush the chicken breasts with olive oil.

3. Grill each side of the chicken breasts for 2–3 minutes then place them on a baking tray, cover with foil, and cook in the oven for another 15 minutes or until cooked through.

4. Make the dressing by placing the berries, vinegar, and apple juice concentrate in a small saucepan and heating gently for 3 minutes. Blend in a food processor and set aside to cool.

5. Lay the lettuce on a serving plate and arrange the avocado, fennel, and celery on top.

6. Slice the chicken and lay it over the salad with the snow pea sprouts and pomegranate seeds over the top.

7. Dress with the raspberry vinaigrette and serve immediately.

SALSAS AND SAUCES

With a few basic salsas and sauces up your sleeve you can create really interesting dishes with some very plain ingredients.

OLIVE, CILANTRO, TOMATO, CHILI, AND LIME SALSA

Serves 4–6

Take a piece of lean meat, brush it lightly with olive oil, grill it, and serve it under this salsa, and with very little effort you'll create a delicious meal that's full of flavor and packed with nutrients.

6 large vine-ripened tomatoes

½ red onion, peeled and finely chopped

1 small red chili, seeded and finely chopped

½ cup pitted kalamata olives, finely chopped

½ bunch cilantro (leaves only), roughly chopped

juice of 2 limes

black pepper

METHOD

1. Using a sharp knife, cut a small cross in the bottom of each tomato. Soak the tomatoes in boiling water until the skin starts to crack and peel. Remove the tomatoes from the boiling water with a slotted spoon. Allow them to cool a little so you don't burn yourself, then skin the tomatoes completely. Slice tomatoes in half, remove the seeds, and chop the flesh finely.

2. Combine the tomatoes with the onion, chili, olives, and cilantro leaves.

3. Add the lime juice and season with black pepper.

BASIC TOMATO AND BASIL SAUCE

Makes 4 cups

The trick to a good pasta sauce is the time taken to cook it — rushed, the sauce will be bitter. There's no need to add sugar when you allow it to simmer slowly for at least 50 minutes. The longer it cooks, the more antioxidants it contains.

3 tablespoons virgin olive oil

1 cup fresh basil, chopped

1 small onion, finely chopped

3 cloves garlic, finely chopped

1 small carrot, finely chopped

1 tablespoon fresh thyme, finely chopped

1 tablespoon fresh oregano, finely chopped

4 14-ounce cans of tomatoes, chopped

METHOD

1. Heat the oil in a large saucepan until it's very hot but not smoking.

2. Add the basil and "deep-fry" for a couple of minutes.

3. Add the onion, garlic, carrot, and herbs and sauté until soft.

4. Add the tomatoes and bring to the boil.

5. Reduce the heat and simmer for 50 minutes or until the liquid has thickened and reduced by half.

Cheat's Tip: *If you're buying pasta sauce, check the ingredients and nutrition facts to find a sauce that's made from fresh ingredients and is low in salt and sugar. There are some great ones around and they are excellent to stash away in the pantry in case of an emergency.*

LIME, CORN, AND CILANTRO SALSA

Serves 4

As befitting its Mexican origin, this Mexican corn-and-lime salsa is as delicious with spicy beans as it is grilled chicken or fish.

2 cobs sweet corn

juice of 2 limes

1 small red onion, peeled and finely chopped

½ cup cilantro leaves, chopped

1 red chili, seeded and finely chopped

METHOD

1. Steam the corn cobs for 3 minutes.

2. Once cool, remove the kernels from the cob.

3. Mix the lime juice, red onion, cilantro leaves, chili, and corn kernels together in a bowl.

4. Allow the flavors to combine for at least 1 hour before serving.

WALNUT PESTO

Makes ½ cup

This walnut pesto uses fennel in place of Parmesan and has cayenne for an extra kick. It's delicious served over grilled fish or chicken and mashed pumpkin, or with slow-roasted tomatoes and pasta.

3 tablespoons raw walnuts, chopped

1 bunch flat-leaf parsley

½ cup basil leaves

2 cloves garlic, chopped

1 small piece of fennel, chopped (to make approximately 2 tablespoons)

1 pinch cayenne pepper

juice of ½ lemon

a pinch sea salt

⅓ cup extra-virgin olive oil

METHOD

1. Dry-roast the walnuts in a small, flat pan over a medium heat until they have toasted and turned golden brown, approximately 3–4 minutes.

2. In a food processor, place the walnuts, parsley, basil leaves, garlic, fennel, cayenne pepper, lemon juice, and sea salt.

3. Process the ingredients, adding the olive oil slowly while the motor is running until the pesto is well combined but not completely smooth. The pesto should still have a granular texture.

4. Store ready for use in the refrigerator in an airtight jar.

Notes: *Half a teaspoon of an herb or spice can transform a dish from bland to inspiring. An investment in a few excellent quality herbs and spices is well worth it. To ensure quality and freshness, find a shop with high turnover of products or, better still, a specialty spice store. To retain freshness, spices should always be stored in airtight containers away from sunlight.*

SIDE DISHES

The title "side dish" is not intended to give the impression that these dishes are less important than any of the others. Here you will find a collection of delicious and extremely healthy accessories to dress up the simplest meal. Many may take center stage in front of the grilled meat or fish they are served with.

STIR-FRIED ASIAN GREENS

Serves 4

Try not to let a single day go by without eating a serving of leafy green vegetables. Here's a very fast and easy way to serve Asian greens. There's no need
to follow the ingredients to the letter here — any variety of greens will work,
but try to vary the look and texture to make the dish interesting.

> 2 tablespoons white sesame seeds
>
> 1 bunch broccolini
>
> 2 cups snow peas
>
> 1 bunch bok choy
>
> ½ bunch shallots
>
> ½ tablespoon sesame oil
>
> 1 tablespoon tamari
>
> 2 teaspoons lemon juice
>
> 1 piece fresh ginger, grated (approximately ¾ inch)
>
> 2 cloves garlic, chopped
>
> 1 tablespoon olive oil

METHOD

1. Dry-roast the sesame seeds in a small pan over medium
   heat until golden.

2. Wash the greens and trim them to pieces of similar
   length.

3. Mix the sesame oil, tamari, lemon juice, ginger, and garlic
   in a small bowl.

4. In a wok heat the olive oil until hot, add the broccolini,
   and cook for approximately 1 minute.

5. Add the remaining greens and toss the dressing in at the
   same time.

6. Cook for another 2 minutes.

7. Serve on a platter with sesame seeds sprinkled over the top.

LENTIL DAHL

Serves 4

It may seem like cheap peasant food, but you'll be surprised how enjoyable and satisfying dahl is if you haven't had it before. Lentils are much easier to digest than legumes (beans) and, unlike beans, don't require any soaking.

1 tablespoon olive oil

1 onion, peeled and finely chopped

1 large red bell pepper, finely chopped

2 cloves garlic, crushed

1 tablespoon fresh ginger, peeled and grated

½ teaspoon ground ginger

1 teaspoon allspice

½ teaspoon chili flakes

½ teaspoon ground cloves

1½ cups red lentils, rinsed and drained

2 fresh bay leaves

1 cup water

3 cups vegetable stock

METHOD

1. Heat the olive oil in a medium-sized saucepan.

2. Add the onion, bell pepper, garlic, fresh ginger, and ground spices and sauté for 3–4 minutes.

3. Add the lentils, bay leaves, water, and vegetable stock and bring to a boil.

4. Reduce the heat and simmer partially covered for 40 minutes until the lentils are tender and most of the liquid is absorbed.

5. Serve with cucumber, yogurt-and-mint dip, steamed greens, and a grain.

Note: *To complete the protein and make all eight essential amino acids, lentils should be served with a grain. Rice or chapatis are the traditional accompaniments to dahl. If you do want to use rice, use brown rice.*

"BETTER THAN MASH" BARLEY AND BEAN POT

Serves 4

There are plenty of things to serve with a meal other than mashed potatoes and boiled rice. This barley and bean pot is delicious served with grilled lamb, chicken (see recipe for Barbecued Chicken with Preserved Lemon on page 224), or fish.

1 cup pearl barley

2 cups water

2 cups chicken stock

2 cups green beans, trimmed and cut in half lengthwise

METHOD

1. Rinse the barley thoroughly in cold water.

2. In a medium-sized pan, add the barley, water, and stock and bring to a boil. Reduce the heat and simmer uncovered for 40 minutes, stirring occasionally, until the grain is soft and most of the liquid has absorbed into the grain.

3. Add the beans and cook for another 5 minutes.

BARBECUED CORN WITH LEMON-INFUSED OLIVE OIL

Serves 4

Flavored olive oils are becoming increasingly popular and are available from most good delis. If you can't find any flavored oils, simply combine fresh lemon juice with olive oil in the ratio of 1 to 3.

4 whole sweet corns cob with the husks on

2 tablespoons lemon-infused olive oil

cracked black pepper

METHOD

1. Soak the cobs in water for about 5 minutes.

2. Lay the corn on an oiled griddle and cook the cobs for 15–20 minutes, turning regularly to prevent the husks from becoming too brown.

3. Strip back the husks, leaving them on the cob to be used as a handle. Drizzle with lemon-infused olive oil, sprinkle with black pepper, and serve.

GARLIC AND CHICKPEA MASH

Serves 4

With a good food processor, you'll soon come to love using beans and chickpeas as a replacement for potatoes and rice. Here we mix chickpeas with roasted garlic to pack an even bigger nutritional punch.

½ bulb garlic (skin left on)

1 14-ounce can chickpeas, drained and rinsed

1 tablespoon olive oil

1 teaspoon chili oil

½ cup finely chopped parsley

sea salt and black pepper

METHOD

1. Preheat the oven to 350°F.

2. Place the garlic on a small tray in the oven to roast for 25 minutes or until soft.

3. Peel the garlic and squeeze it into a food processor. Add the chickpeas and process for 1–2 minutes.

4. Add the oils and continue to process until smooth.

5. Stir in the chopped parsley and season to taste.

6. Serve warm under grilled lamb or as a spread in sandwiches.

CRACKED SWEET-AND-SOUR FREEKEH

Serves 4

Forget the gloopy sauce used to make sweet-and-sour dishes in Chinese restaurants. The combination of prunes and preserved lemons is delicious with freekeh. This salad can be served as an accompaniment to barbecued chicken or roast duck.

1 cup cracked freekeh

8 pitted prunes, finely chopped

2 preserved lemons, flesh removed and discarded and skin finely chopped

1 cup Italian parsley, finely chopped

cracked black pepper

a pinch sea salt

METHOD

1. Cook the freekeh as per instructions on the packet.

2. While still warm, combine with remaining ingredients and serve.

SPICY RED CABBAGE WITH CRANBERRIES

Serves 6

Red cabbage and cranberries for a multitude of antioxidants, spices to boost the metabolism and aid digestion, and a wonderful fusion of flavors make this variation on a traditional German dish an excellent companion to turkey, duck, or chicken.

1 tablespoon corn oil

1 red onion, finely chopped

2 cloves garlic, crushed

½ teaspoon cinnamon

½ teaspoon ground nutmeg

½ tablespoon grated fresh ginger

½ red cabbage, thinly sliced

1½ tablespoons apple cider vinegar

2 tablespoons apple juice concentrate

½ cup frozen cranberries

METHOD

1. Heat the oil in a heavy pan.

2. Add the onion and garlic and sauté for 2 minutes.

3. Add the spices, cabbage, vinegar, and apple juice concentrate and stir.

4. Reduce the heat to low and cover the pan.

5. Cook for 20 minutes.

6. Add the cranberries, stir, and cook for another 15 minutes.

BRUSSELS SPROUTS WITH ROASTED PINE NUT AND LEMON MUSTARD DRESSING

Serves 4

Anyone who's eaten overcooked Brussels sprouts will never want to eat them again. Fear and loathing is the common complaint made against these poor, misunderstood greens. Brussels sprouts must be cooked through — neither too crisp nor gray and mushy. Select sprouts of similar size and test them with a small, sharp knife after 5 minutes and every minute thereafter.

24 medium-sized Brussels sprouts

¼ cup pine nuts

1½ tablespoons olive oil

juice of ½ lemon

1 teaspoon mustard, without seeds

zest of 1 lemon

METHOD

1. Trim the Brussels sprouts and remove the outer leaves. Using a sharp knife, make a cross incision at the base of each sprout.

2. Dry-roast the pine nuts in a small frying pan over medium heat, taking care not to burn them.

3. Steam the sprouts for approximately 5–7 minutes, depending on their size. Drain thoroughly.

4. In a small saucepan, heat the olive oil and stir in the lemon juice, mustard, and pine nuts.

5. Toss with the sprouts and serve immediately topped with grated lemon zest.

DINNERS

Were we only to eat for health, we'd be best advised to eat the main meal of the day at lunchtime and reserve the smaller meal for the end of the day. In doing so, our food would be well on its way to being digested before we go to bed. Given, however, that the aim is to eat for health and pleasure, and most of us don't have a lifestyle to accommodate leisurely mid-day eating, the main meal of the day will invariably be served in the evening. Make an occasion of the main meal of the day. Sit down at the table, switch off the TV, and take time to enjoy your food while relaxing with your family or friends. And, to ensure a good night's sleep, give yourself a few hours after eating before going to bed.

Meat

It's a personal choice whether to eat meat or not, but after reading the meat section I'm sure you'll agree there's no disputing its value in a healthy diet. The great thing these days is that there are so many lean cuts of meat available. Bear in mind that if you cook lean meat for too long it will turn out tough. Regardless, it's always better to enjoy meat rare or medium rare because overcooked grilled meat produces carcinogens.

CHILI

Serves 4

This is an old favorite of students on a tight budget who need to fill up, heat up, and who don't want to go to a lot of trouble.

Commonly served with rice or on large baked potatoes, chili is better served with quinoa or with extra beans and a large salad.

1 tablespoon olive oil

1 large yellow onion, peeled and finely chopped

2 cloves garlic, peeled and crushed

2 small red chilies, seeded and finely chopped

12 ounces premium lean, ground beef

1 14-ounce can whole tomatoes, chopped

1 tablespoon tomato paste

2 cups beef stock

1 green bell pepper, finely diced

1 14-ounce can kidney beans

METHOD

1. Pour oil into pan and sauté the onion and garlic for 3–4 minutes until soft.

2. Add the chilies and ground beef and cook gently until the beef is evenly browned.

3. Add the tomatoes, tomato paste, beef stock, bell pepper, and kidney beans and bring to a boil.

4. Reduce the heat to a simmer, partially cover the pan, and cook on the stove top for 45 minutes or until the liquid has reduced down to a thick sauce.

Tip: *Chili is good stuffed into halved red bell peppers, covered in foil, and baked in the oven for 20–25 minutes.*

ROLLED BEEF WITH ASPARAGUS AND SHALLOTS

Makes 16 pieces, serves 4

Combining asparagus and shallots, these pretty little rolls make an excellent main dish served with buckwheat noodles or brown sushi rice.

> *8 asparagus stalks*
>
> *8 shallots*
>
> *16 ounces of beef sirloin, beaten with a mallet into 4 very thin sheets*
>
> *2 tablespoons grapeseed oil*
>
> *1½ ounces sake*
>
> *½ tablespoon rice syrup*
>
> *1½ tablespoons mirin*
>
> *2 tablespoons reduced-sodium soy sauce*
>
> *wasabi, to serve*

Note: *Sake is an alcoholic Japanese rice wine available from Asian stores. While there are some reports suggesting sake has numerous health benefits, like all other alcoholic beverages it should be consumed in moderation. It also contains no sulphites — the chemicals found in white wine and dried fruit that can cause asthma-like symptoms in some people. When cooking with alcohol, the alcohol content is burned off.*

METHOD

1. Break the ends off the asparagus, and cut the stalks in half.

2. Trim the shallots at the roots and cut them to the length of the asparagus.

3. Place the asparagus and shallots in a steamer for 2–3 minutes until the asparagus is tender.

4. Rinse with cold water.

5. Spread beef slices on a board, and lay two asparagus and shallot pieces onto each piece of meat.

6. Roll the beef around the vegetables and trim the ends.

7. Heat oil in a frying pan and brown the rolls.

8. Remove from the pan and set aside.

9. Combine the sake, rice syrup, mirin, and soy sauce in the frying pan and cook for 5–6 minutes to reduce.

10. Return the beef rolls to the pan and toss around to coat with the sauce.

11. Cut the rolls into pieces about 1 inch wide and arrange in a serving dish.

12. Serve with wasabi.

BEEF FILLET WITH SALSA VERDE

Serves 4

The translation of salsa verde is green sauce, which is probably why we've adopted the Italian name. It has a strong taste and is delicious on full-flavored fish like mackerel and tuna as well as red meat.

4 fillets of beef (approximately 7 ounces each)

Salsa verde

1 cup curly parsley

1 cup flat-leaf parsley

2 cloves garlic, crushed

¼ cup capers, rinsed and drained

2 teaspoons creamy horseradish

juice of 1 large lemon

¼ cup olive oil

ground black pepper

METHOD

1. To make the salsa verde, put the parsley, garlic, capers, horseradish, and lemon in a food processor and process until combined.

2. Slowly add the olive oil and process until the sauce has a consistent texture. Season with black pepper.

3. Brush the steaks with olive oil and set aside.

4. Heat a grill pan and cook the steaks for 3–5 minutes on each side, depending on how you like your steak cooked.

5. Serve with the salsa verde on top.

MARINATED LAMB AND VEGETABLE KEBABS

Serves 4

Even though there is less saturated fat on trimmed cuts of meat, there is and never has been any fiber. Are the high incidents of colon cancer a result of too much meat or not enough vegetables? There is much research to suggest the latter. So, whenever you have a meat dish, do as we have done in this dish and incorporate several extra veggies.

¼ cup olive oil

1 tablespoon honey

2 cloves garlic

juice of 1 large lemon

1 tablespoon mint, chopped

1 tablespoon rosemary leaves, chopped

1 red chili, finely chopped

black pepper, to season

9 ounces button mushrooms, cleaned

1 red onion, chopped into wedges

3 baby eggplant, chopped into ¾-inch pieces

3 zucchini, chopped into ¾-inch pieces

18 ounces trimmed lamb, diced

METHOD

1. Combine the olive oil with the honey, garlic, lemon juice, herbs, chili, and pepper in a small bowl.

2. Pour the marinade over the lamb and set aside to marinate for at least 30 minutes.

3. Thread the lamb and vegetables onto pre-soaked bamboo skewers, reserving the marinade to baste.

4. Seal the meat under a hot grill or on a hotplate for 3–4 minutes, turning and basting with reserved marinade occasionally.

5. Reduce the heat and cook for another 3–4 minutes for medium or 4–5 minutes for well-done lamb.

HEALTHY HARIRA

Serves 4

This delicious Moroccan lamb dish has the double bonus of two fabulous carbs — barley and lentils. It makes a hearty mid-week meal in winter and tastes even better as leftovers.

1 tablespoon olive oil

9 ounces lean lamb, cut into cubes

1 yellow onion, peeled and chopped

1 pinch saffron threads

½ teaspoon cinnamon

½ teaspoon ground turmeric

¾ teaspoon ground ginger

2 tablespoons pearl barley

6 cups vegetable stock

½ cup green lentils

2 14-ounce cans tomatoes

1 tablespoon tomato paste (no sugar or salt added)

1 red bell pepper, seeded and chopped

1 bunch cilantro leaves, roughly chopped

juice of 1 lemon

sea salt and black pepper

METHOD

1. Heat the oil in a large, heavy pan, add the lamb, and fry for about 2 minutes until the pieces are brown.

2. Add the onion and spices and cook until the onion is soft.

3. Add the barley and stock and bring to a boil.

4. Reduce to simmer and cook for 30 minutes.

5.   Add the lentils, tomatoes, tomato paste, and bell pepper and cook for another 30 minutes until the lentils are tender.

6. Stir in the cilantro and lemon juice just before serving and season to taste.

GRILLED CHICKEN WITH SMOKED PAPRIKA, CHILI, AND BELL PEPPER SAUCE

Serves 4

The sauce in this dish can be used in any variety of ways other than with grilled chicken. It's delicious over grilled lamb, lentil burgers, and even as a dip with vegetable crudités.

1 red bell pepper

2 large red chili peppers

4 small organic chicken breasts

olive oil

1 small red chili, seeded and finely chopped

juice of ½ lemon

½ teaspoon smoked paprika

pinch sea salt

METHOD

1. Preheat the oven to 350°F.

2. Grill the bell pepper and chili peppers until they have blackened all over.

3. Remove from the grill and put them in a plastic bag to release the skins.

4. Brush the chicken with olive oil and grill on each side for 2–3 minutes.

5. Transfer to a baking tray and place in the oven to cook through for 15 minutes.

6. Peel the skin from the bell pepper and chili peppers and put the flesh in a food processor.

7. Add the chili, lemon juice, paprika, and seasoning and process until it's smooth.

8. Serve over grilled chicken with steamed greens.

CHICKEN AND TOMATO BAKE

Serves 4

We've snuck in a little grated Parmesan to give the quinoa a slightly golden crust and sharper flavor. Although the cheese is saturated fat, a little goes a long way when it's grated.

1¼ pounds organic chicken breasts

1½ cups tomato and basil sauce (see recipe, page 197)

1 cup quinoa

2 cups water

¼ cup grated Parmesan

1 bunch spinach

METHOD

1. Preheat oven to 350°F.

2. Cut the chicken into strips approximately ½ inch thick.

3. Arrange them in a baking dish and cover with a layer of tomato and basil sauce. Cover with foil and bake for 20–25 minutes.

4. Add the quinoa to the water and bring to a boil.

5. Cover the pan and reduce to simmer for 15 minutes until the water is completely absorbed and the quinoa is soft.

6. Stir the Parmesan through the quinoa.

7. Top the chicken and tomato and basil sauce with the quinoa and Parmesan mix, and return to the oven for another 10 minutes.

8. Steam the spinach for 3 minutes.

9. Remove chicken bake from the oven and serve immediately with the spinach.

BARBECUED CHICKEN
WITH PRESERVED LEMON

Serves 4

Preserved lemon is made with lemon juice and a lot of salt, which of course is not a big plus when it comes to good health. If, however, your diet is relatively free of packaged food products and you don't add salt to your food, automatically you are eating less salt than the average person. That's my justification anyway to include a small amount of this wonderful condiment in your cooking. When using preserved lemons, discard the fleshy pulp and use the peel only.

4 pieces preserved lemon

2 tablespoons lemon juice

2 cloves garlic

1 teaspoon ground cumin

1 teaspoon sweet paprika

⅓ cup olive oil

cracked black pepper

¼ bunch cilantro leaves, roughly chopped

2 cilantro roots, washed

4 organic chicken breasts

METHOD

1. Remove the pulp from the preserved lemon and add the rind to a food processor with the lemon juice, garlic, cumin, paprika, oil, pepper, and the cilantro leaves and roots and process until smooth.

2. Wipe the chicken breasts with damp paper towel to clean and smear the marinade over each of them.

3. Set aside to marinate in the refrigerator for 1–2 hours.

4. Preheat barbecue grill.

5. Cook chicken on the barbecue for approximately 7 minutes each side, turning once.

Fish

Fish is one of the healthiest sources of protein available. It's rich in omega-3 fatty acids, low in saturated fat, and is easy to prepare and cook. Buy it fresh and cook it on the day of buying, and buy American rather than imported when possible. Approximately three-quarters of the world's oceans are fished up to their limits with as much as 90 percent of the large predatory fish such as bluefin tuna, shark, and swordfish lost. These fish also have a higher concentration of mercury and are best avoided (see page 61 for more information) to preserve both our ecosystem and our health.

BARLEY AND PEA RISOTTO
WITH GRILLED SALMON

Serves 4

While it doesn't have the creamy consistency of rice risotto, this barley risotto is just as comforting with many more health benefits. Once you get used to making risotto with barley, there's no going back.

2 large cloves garlic, crushed

1 tablespoon olive oil

3 cups fish stock

1 cup pearl barley, rinsed

4 salmon fillets, skin left on

olive oil, extra

juice of 1 lime

freshly ground black pepper

2 shallots, finely chopped

1 cup fresh shelled peas

½ cup chervil, chopped

METHOD

1. Preheat the oven to 350°F.

2. Sauté the garlic and olive oil in a heavy, oven-proof dish for 2 minutes. Add the fish stock and gently bring it to a boil.

3. Add the barley, cover the pan with a lid, and transfer it to the middle shelf of the oven for 50 minutes.

4. After the barley has been cooking for approximately 40 minutes, brush the salmon fillets with olive oil and lime juice and season with black pepper.

5. Heat an oiled grill pan and sear the salmon on the skin side for 2 minutes. Turn and sear on the other side for another minute. Remove from the heat and set aside.

6. Remove the barley risotto from the oven, add the shallots and peas, then lay the fish on top.

7. Return to the oven for 10 minutes.

8. Remove from the oven, sprinkle the chervil on top, and serve with a green salad.

GRILLED SNAPPER FILLET WITH BULGUR, PARSLEY, AND ROASTED ALMONDS

Serves 4

Served with a chili and bell pepper sauce (see page 221), this meal tastes and looks stunning.

1 cup bulgur

2 cups water

¼ cup almonds, dry-roasted in a pan and roughly chopped

½ cup flat-leaf parsley, chopped

4 snapper fillets

olive oil for brushing

1 tablespoon lemon juice

cracked black pepper

METHOD

1. Preheat the oven to 400°F.

2. Soak the bulgur in 2 cups boiling water for 30 minutes.

3. Squeeze any excess moisture from the soaked bulgur and mix in the roasted almonds and chopped parsley.

4. Brush the snapper with a little olive oil, lemon juice, and black pepper and grill for 5 minutes each side.

5. Serve the snapper over the bulgur with chili and black pepper sauce and a green salad.

BAKED COD WITH EGGPLANT, BELL PEPPER, AND LIMA BEANS

Serves 4

If cod is unavailable, try any other firm-fleshed white fish like snapper.

¼ cup olive oil

2 medium eggplant, cut into 1-inch cubes

3 large vine-ripened tomatoes, diced

2 red bell peppers cut into strips

1 small red chili

4 cloves garlic, crushed

4 cod fillets

olive oil, to brush fish

lemon juice, to brush fish

1 can lima beans, drained

cracked black pepper

sea salt

METHOD

1. Preheat oven to 350°F.

2. Heat the oil in a baking tray until hot. Remove from the oven and add the eggplant, tomato, bell pepper, chili, and garlic.

3. Toss so the olive oil is covering all the vegetables and return to the oven to cook for 10 minutes.

4. While the veggies are cooking, brush the cod with a little olive oil and lemon juice and sear in a nonstick pan for 1–2 minutes on each side. Then lay the fish on a separate tray lined with parchment paper and cook for another 10 minutes in the oven.

5. Remove the veggies from the oven, add the lima beans, and gently toss. Season with salt and pepper.

6. Place the veggie mixture on serving plates. Top with the cooked fish. Serve with steamed greens.

RUBY RED TROUT

Serves 4

The combination of grapefruit and tomatoes with the trout is superb and looks particularly magnificent served with chard and olive oil.

2 ruby red grapefruit, segmented

½ cup mint

4 roma tomatoes, seeded

1 tablespoon extra-virgin olive oil

1 clove garlic, crushed

cracked black pepper

4 trout fillets

METHOD

1. Slice between the membranes of the ruby red grapefruits to remove the pith.

2. Finely slice the mint and dice the ripe roma tomatoes.

3. Warm the olive oil in a pan, add the garlic, tomatoes, and cracked pepper and simmer for 5 minutes.

4. Add the mint and grapefruit segments and continue to simmer with the juice from the grapefruit.

5. While the sauce is cooking, grill the trout for approximately 3–5 minutes on each side, depending on how you like it cooked.

6. Lay the vegetable and grapefruit mix on serving plates and arrange the cooked trout on top.

GRILLED COD WITH SAGE, LENTILS, AND ROASTED BELL PEPPER

Serves 2

Lentils combined with preserved limes and roasted bell pepper make a delicious base to this easy fish dish.

2 cod fillets (approximately 5 ounces each)

½ tablespoon olive oil

1 tablespoon olive oil, extra

juice of ½ lemon

1 tablespoon capers, rinsed and drained

½ bunch sage leaves

1 can lentils, drained and rinsed

2 preserved limes, flesh scraped and discarded, rind finely chopped

1 prepared roasted bell pepper, sliced

METHOD

1. Preheat the oven to 350°F.

2. Wipe the fish with a damp cloth.

3. Make a few incisions across the thickest part of the fillets and brush with ½ tablespoon olive oil and lemon juice.

4. Heat the extra olive oil until hot but not smoking and add the capers and sage leaves. Cook until they're crispy.

5. Remove from the oil and lay them out on absorbent paper towel to drain them of excess oil.

6. Heat a grill pan and sear the fish for 2 minutes on each side, then transfer the fish to a baking tray and cook in the oven for 15–20 minutes to cook through.

7. While the fish is cooking, heat the lentils in a pan and stir through the preserved limes and bell pepper.

8. When the fish is cooked, sprinkle the capers and sage through the lentils.

9. Serve fish on top of the lentils with an accompanying green salad.

POACHED TROUT WITH GREEN TEA SALSA

Serves 4

It's not often you can serve up a meal with as unique as this dish. The green tea salsa served with trout poached in green tea is absolutely delicious and very different — and, of course, it has numerous health benefits.

4 tablespoons sencha tea

6 cups boiling water

4 skinless trout fillets

1 bunch cilantro leaves

3 cilantro roots, scraped clean

½ cup flat-leaf parsley

¼ cup extra-virgin camellia tea oil

1 tablespoon green tea leaves

juice of 1 lime

3 anchovy fillets, drained of oil

black pepper

1 bunch bok choy

METHOD

1. Place the sencha tea leaves in a pan with the water and steep for five minutes. Strain the leaves and return the tea to the pan.

2. Place the trout fillets into the pan, making sure they are completely covered in tea and bring the tea back to a boil over moderate heat. As soon as the tea starts to boil, turn off the heat and cover the pan. Leave the trout to sit in the water for approximately 1 hour.

3. Place the cilantro leaves and roots, parsley, camellia oil, green tea leaves, lime juice, anchovies, and black pepper into a food processor and process until smooth.

4. Strain the trout and serve with the salsa on top and accompanied by steamed bok choy.

BAKED MACKEREL AND MUSHROOMS

Serves 4

The "freedom with fish club" is one that you'll automatically join when you realize there are few boundaries when serving fish. With the technique of cooking fish down pat, you will quickly learn that, like meat, it can be combined with any vegetable, served with a multitude of sauces, and laid on top of anything you would lay a piece of steak on. Here we combine the delicate flavors of various mushrooms with one of our favorite fish, mackerel.

¼ cup olive oil

2 cloves garlic, crushed

14 ounces mixed mushrooms, chopped (brown, shiitake, oyster, button)

1 cup fish stock

pinch sea salt

cracked black pepper

4 mackerel fillets

olive oil for brushing fish

½ bunch flat-leaf parsley

METHOD

1. Preheat the oven to 400°F.

2. Heat the oil in a pan and add the garlic and mushrooms. Cook over medium heat for about 4 minutes.

3. Add the stock and the seasoning, simmer for another 4 minutes, and set aside.

4. Brush the fillets with olive oil. Heat a nonstick pan and sear the fish (skin side first) for 1 minute. Turn it over and sear the other side for 30 seconds.

5. Transfer the fish to a baking tray and place in the oven for 3–4 minutes.

6. Gently reheat the mushrooms and add the parsley.

7. Serve the fish on top of a bed of mushrooms and accompany the dish with some lightly steamed spinach.

Note: *Many fish can easily turn from succulent and moist to bone dry when cooked. Take care not to overcook it.*

MACKEREL WITH PINE NUTS AND CUCUMBER AND LEMON SALSA

Serves 4

½ cup pine nuts

2 tablespoons fresh rosemary leaves

4 mackerel fillets (approximately 5 ounces each)

Salsa

2 Persian cucumbers

juice of 1 lemon

2 segments of preserved lemon peel, finely chopped

1 tablespoon chopped mint

METHOD

1. To make the salsa, thinly slice the cucumber using a potato peeler.

2. Place the slices in a nonreactive bowl and add the lemon juice, preserved lemon, and mint. Mix it all together and rest a plate over the surface to weigh the ingredients down.

3. Chill in the refrigerator for 2–3 hours.

4. To prepare the remainder of the dish, grind the pine nuts and rosemary together in a spice grinder.

5. Press the mixture over each side of the fish with the flat blade of a knife. Cover the grill pan with foil and grill the fish over moderate heat for 4 minutes each side, taking care not to burn the pine nuts.

6. Serve with the cucumber and lemon salsa and steamed spinach.

VEGETARIAN DISHES

Not so many years ago, a meal devoid of meat was incomplete and only enjoyed by unshaven weirdos! Fortunately, this closed mentality is now a thing of the past and the mainstream finally recognizes that many vegetarian dishes are more creative, beautiful, and delicious than those using meat, poultry, or fish can ever be.

GREEN TEA BARLEY RISOTTO WITH MUSHROOMS AND ASPARAGUS

Serves 4

Genmaicha is a Japanese green tea blended with toasted brown rice. It's available from most Asian grocers and is popular with many who don't like the strong flavor of green tea. Used in this barley risotto, it makes a delicious, nutty, and nourishing low-GI meal the whole family will enjoy. To boost protein, serve the risotto under a piece of white fish steamed in ginger and light soy sauce.

3 tablespoons camellia tea oil

7 ounces brown mushrooms, finely sliced

3½ ounces shiitake mushrooms, finely sliced

2 cloves garlic, crushed

½ tablespoon grated fresh ginger

1 cup pearl barley

2½ cups genmaicha tea, strained

1 tablespoon tamari

10 asparagus stalks, trimmed and cut in half

5 shallots, finely sliced

2 limes

METHOD

1. Heat the oil in a heavy pan. Sauté the mushrooms with the garlic and ginger for approximately five minutes.

2. Add the barley and stir to coat the grains with oil.

3. Add the genmaicha and tamari and slowly bring to a boil.

4. Reduce to a simmer, stir, and cover the pan to cook for 1 hour. Check occasionally that the grain is not sticking to the bottom of the pan and add a little extra genmaicha if necessary.

5. Add the asparagus and shallots in the final 2 minutes of cooking.

6. Serve with sliced fresh limes over the risotto.

SPRING VEGGIE PIE

Serves 6

There's something so fulfilling about making a pie from scratch and it is so satisfying to sit down to eat. This rustic pie takes a little time but is very easy and enjoyable to make — particularly when it's designed to look imperfect! The true perfectionists may want to cook their own lentils, but canned work just as well and remove a step from this labor of love.

Poppy Seed Pastry

1 cup whole-wheat spelt flour

¾ cup white spelt flour

pinch sea salt

1 tablespoon poppy seeds

⅓ cup omega spread (see notes)

¼ cup cold ice water

Filling

1 tablespoon olive oil

9 ounces pumpkin, peeled

3 cloves garlic

1 tablespoon rosemary

9 ounces mushrooms

7 ounces green beans, trimmed and cut into pieces approximately 1-inch long

1 14-ounce can lentils, drained and rinsed

2 tablespoons shiromiso (white miso)

⅓ cup water

METHOD

1. To make the pastry, place the flours, seasoning, omega spread, and poppy seeds in a food processor.

2. Process until well combined.

3. Slowly add the ice water while the processor is still on until the dough is stiff enough to form a ball.

4. Place the dough in the refrigerator for 20–25 minutes.

5. Preheat the oven to 350°F.

6. To make the filling, heat the olive oil in a baking tray and, once hot, add the pumpkin, garlic, rosemary, and mushrooms. Toss and place in the oven to roast for 15–20 minutes.

7. Steam the green beans for 4 minutes then drain and rinse in cold water.

8. Mix the roasted veggies, lentils, and green beans together and set aside to cool.

9. Mix the shiromiso with water to make a smooth paste and combine in the bowl with the lentils, roasted veggies, and beans.

10. Roll the pastry out and place on a pizza stone or lined baking tray.

11. Fill the middle of the pastry with the lentils and veggies then fold it up and over the edges to form a rustic-looking pie.

12. Bake in the oven for 20–25 minutes.

Notes: *Frozen, prerolled pastry is likely to contain trans fats, known to reduce levels of protective (HDL) cholesterol while increasing levels of harmful (LDL) cholesterol.*

Omega spread is available from health food stores and is made from a blend of omega-3 and omega-6 fatty acids using a cold process which does not involve hydrogenation. It contains no trans fats or cholesterol.

CHARD, PUMPKIN, AND PINE NUT ROLL

Serves 4

This dish looks far more complicated than it actually is and tastes really delicious.

1 bunch chard, washed and stalks removed

½ teaspoon nutmeg

sea salt and pepper

2–3 cups pumpkin, peeled and cut into chunks

6 egg whites

3½ ounces soft goat cheese

1 tablespoon pine nuts, roasted

METHOD

1. Preheat the oven to 350°F.

2. Cook the chard in boiling water for 2 minutes. Plunge into cold water and squeeze dry.

3. Blend the chard in a food processor with nutmeg and seasoning.

4. Brush the pumpkin with a little olive oil and sprinkle with a little sea salt and pepper and place on a baking tray. Place in the oven to bake for 20 minutes.

5. Beat the egg whites until stiff peaks form.

6. Gently fold the chard through the egg whites, taking care not to overbeat them.

7. Line a baking sheet with baking paper and spread the egg white mixture over the tray. Place in the oven to cook for 10 minutes until it's cooked through but still soft and springy. Remove from oven and ease gently from the tray with a flat knife and spatula and lay it out on a clean tea towel.

8. Spread the goat cheese over the egg white base and sprinkle the pine nuts on top.

9. Lay the roast pumpkin over the top of the pine nuts mashing it down gently with a fork.

10. Using the tea towel to guide you, roll it up and serve with a fresh green salad.

SAUTÉED CHARD, OLIVE, AND FENNEL PASTA

Serves 4

There are some things you should have in the refrigerator and pantry at all times like a good-quality Parmesan (a little of it goes a long way so don't worry about the fat content), some kalamata olives, olive oil, whole-wheat pasta, and garlic. A quick dash to the store to grab a bunch of spinach and fennel bulbs, and this mid-week dish can be on the table in minutes.

1 pound whole-wheat pasta

1 bunch chard, washed and trimmed

1 tablespoon olive oil

2 cloves garlic, finely sliced

1 fennel bulb, thinly sliced

⅓ cup kalamata olives

2 tablespoons grated Parmesan

black pepper

METHOD

1. Cook the pasta in plenty of boiling water for about 15–20 minutes until it's soft but retains "bite."

2. Cook the chard for 1 minute in plenty of boiling water. Drain thoroughly. Heat the olive oil in a large pan and cook the garlic until golden.

3. Add the fennel and cook for another 3–5 minutes. Toss with the chard and cook for another 2 minutes. Remove from the heat and add the olives.

4. Serve the chard mixture over the pasta. Top with a small amount of grated Parmesan and black pepper.

TOFU, BROCCOLI, AND SESAME STIR-FRY

Serves 2

13 ounces organic firm tofu (cut into cubes)

1 tablespoon sesame oil

1 tablespoon olive oil

1 red bell pepper, cut into strips

1 large red chili, cut into fine strips

14 ounces broccoli (cut into small florets)

1 tablespoon sesame seeds

Sesame Sauce

2 tablespoons unhulled tahini

1 tablespoon mirin

1 tablespoon reduced-sodium tamari

juice of ¼ lemon

juice of a ¾-inch piece of grated ginger root

water

METHOD

1. To make the sesame sauce, mix the tahini with the mirin, tamari, lemon juice, and ginger juice. Add water until it reaches a smooth, creamy consistency.

2. To make the remainder of the dish, bring a medium-sized pan of water to a boil. Add the tofu cubes and return to a boil. Boil until the tofu cubes float to the surface of the water. Drain and blot dry.

3. Heat the sesame oil in a wok and stir-fry the tofu until it becomes slightly golden. Set aside to keep warm.

—101 Healthiest Foods —

4. Heat the olive oil and stir-fry the bell pepper and chili for 2 minutes.

5. Add the broccoli florets and cook for another 3 minutes, adding a little water if required.

6. Remove from the heat. Stir in the tofu and the sesame seeds. Drizzle with the sesame sauce or serve it as a dipping sauce on the side.

Note: *If you don't have a gas oven, it may be worth investing in an electric wok. Electric stoves can't heat woks to high-enough temperatures for stir-frying.*

CHARD, RICOTTA, AND VEGETABLE FRITTATA

Serves 4–6

Perhaps because they're so readily available, eggs generally don't excite the masses. But as anyone who regularly makes frittatas will know, everyone enjoys them.

2 bell peppers

1 onion, finely sliced

1 teaspoon olive oil

1 bunch chard, stalks removed, cut into small pieces

9 ounces low-fat ricotta

¼ cup pickled gherkins, finely chopped

sea salt and cracked pepper

6 free-range eggs

METHOD

1. Preheat the oven to 350°F.

2. Roast the bell peppers in the oven until the skin is burned and blistered. Set aside in a covered container until cool enough to remove the skin and seeds.

3. While the bell pepper is roasting, fry the onion in the olive oil until golden and slightly crispy (approximately 10 minutes).

4. Blanch the chard in boiling water for 2 minutes, drain, and squeeze any excess moisture from it and set aside. Combine the chard with the ricotta and gherkins, season with black pepper and a pinch of sea salt.

5. Separate the egg whites and beat them until they form stiff peaks. Beat the egg yolks in a separate bowl then fold them into the egg white mixture.

6. Lightly grease a 2-quart, oven-proof casserole dish with olive oil. Pour half the egg mixture into the bottom of the dish, then layer the onions and bell pepper over the surface. Spread the chard and ricotta mixture and then top with the remaining egg.

7. Cook in the center of the oven for 20–25 minutes or until set. Serve with a green salad.

SWEET THINGS

We all enjoy a sweet treat now and again, and there are ways of indulging your senses without eating too many unhealthy foods. Making your own treats gets you halfway there because you can ensure the use of good-quality ingredients without added undesirable extras. Here's a few of our favorites incorporating many of our 5-star foods.

RHUBARB AND GINGER NUT CRUMBLE

Serves 6

With this crumble topping, you could replace the rhubarb with pears, raspberries, or any other fruit in season. The topping is much healthier than the traditional crumble made from flour, sugar, and butter — and far tastier! Dry-roast the nuts and seeds in a pan over medium heat until they are toasty, but be careful not to burn them.

1 bunch rhubarb, trimmed

½ cup apple juice concentrate

1 teaspoon grated fresh ginger

¼ cup hazelnuts, dry-roasted

¼ cup almonds, dry-roasted

½ cup rolled oats, dry-roasted

¼ cup sunflower seeds, dry-roasted

¼ cup pepitas (pumpkin seeds), dry-roasted

1 tablespoon sesame seeds, dry-roasted

½ cup barley malt

1 tablespoon almond oil

¼ teaspoon ground cinnamon

METHOD

1. Preheat the oven to 325°F.

2. Wash the rhubarb but don't dry it, and cut into pieces about 1 inch long.

3. Put rhubarb in a pan over low heat, add the apple concentrate and ginger, and cover. The rhubarb will slowly stew in the steam and its own juices.

4. Remove from the heat when the rhubarb is tender but still retains its shape, about 5–10 minutes. Divide rhubarb among 6 individual ramekins and set aside.

5. Coarsely chop the roasted nuts and mix with the oats and seeds.

6. Melt the barley malt in a saucepan with the almond oil and cinnamon and mix with a wooden spoon. Pour the oil and malt mixture over the nut mix and stir until thoroughly combined.

7. Spoon the crumble mixture over the rhubarb and bake for 15 minutes.

SPICY BERRIES WITH VANILLA YOGURT

Serves 6

The chili and herb infusion gives these berries a very interesting flavor.

1 cup water

¼ cup maple syrup

1 vanilla pod, split, with seeds scraped out (reserve the seeds for another use)

½ cup mint leaves, roughly chopped

¼ cup basil leaves, roughly chopped

¼ teaspoon ground chili

12 ounces mixed berries

7 ounces fresh strawberries, washed and hulled

½ teaspoon vanilla extract

7 ounces low-fat natural yogurt

METHOD

1. Heat the water in a pan with the maple syrup and vanilla pod and bring to a boil.

2. Place the herbs in a piece of cheesecloth and tie around with string to make a bag. Drop the bag into the water with the chili.

3. Set aside to cool to room temperature.

4. Pour the liquid over the mixed berries and refrigerate for at least 2 hours.

5. Add the strawberries approximately 1 hour before serving.

6. Stir the vanilla extract into the yogurt and serve with the berries.

HEALTHIER ANZACS

Makes approx. 12 cookies

Anzacs are classic, beloved cookies in Australia and New Zealand. Traditionally, they are hard cookies made with dried coconut and lots of sugar, which gives them a caramel flavor. Still, healthier or not, these anzacs are high in calories and should be enjoyed in moderation.

1 cup rolled oats

¾ cup whole-wheat spelt flour

1 pinch sea salt

¼ cup grapeseed oil

3 tablespoons rice syrup

1 tablespoon boiling water

1 teaspoon baking powder

METHOD

1. Preheat the oven to 375°F.

2. Put the oats into a mixing bowl with the flour and the salt.

3. In a small pan, heat the oil and rice syrup together.

4. In a separate small bowl, add the boiling water to the baking powder.

5. Pour the baking powder and water into the oil and syrup and stir continually while it fizzes up and the liquids combine.

6. Mix the wet ingredients into the dry and combine until the mix forms a ball.

7. Roll the cookie mixture using a rolling pin on a floured surface. Cut the cookies using a cookie cutter.

8. Bake in the oven for 10 minutes.

YOGURT, PISTACHIO, AND FIG CAKES

Serves 4–6

Most of us were brought up to believe that all sweet food is a treat, so it's hard to deny ourselves that pleasure from time to time. The compromise may be to make healthy sweet treats and enjoy them more often than not.

5 dried figs, chopped

2 tablespoons rose water

3 large free range eggs

½ cup honey

12 ounces low-fat yogurt

zest of 1 lemon and ½ orange

juice of ½ lemon

¼ cup coarse semolina

1 ounce pistachios roughly, chopped

METHOD

1. Preheat the oven to 350°F and place a baking tray with boiling water in the oven to stay hot.

2. Soak the figs in rosewater for 15 minutes.

3. Separate the eggs and combine the honey with the egg yolks in a bowl.

4. To the egg yolk mixture, add the yogurt, lemon and orange zest, lemon juice, figs, and semolina and combine well.

5. In a separate bowl, whisk the egg whites until stiff peaks form. Fold the egg yolk mixture into the egg whites.

6. Sprinkle a spoonful of chopped pistachios into the bottom of greased, individual ramekin dishes.

7. Spoon the yogurt mixture into each dish.

8. Place the ramekins into the baking tray (the water should come halfway up the sides of each dish).

9. Bake for 20 minutes or until the top of the spongy cake is light golden on top.

CARROT AND PUMPKIN TEA LOAF

Serves 8

This loaf is a great source of antioxidants and sweet enough to be an enjoyable treat for your kids' play snack, but not too sweet to send them into a sugar-crazed frenzy. With the oil and mashed pumpkin, it will always be moist so don't make the mistake of thinking it's uncooked.

½ cup camellia tea oil

2 free-range eggs

¼ cup honey

1 carrot, finely grated

1 cup mashed pumpkin

1 cup self-raising whole-wheat flour

½ cup walnuts, chopped

½ teaspoon cinnamon

½ teaspoon mixed spice

METHOD

1. Preheat the oven to 350°F.

2. Lightly oil a loaf tin and line the base with parchment paper.

3. Mix the oil, eggs, and honey until well combined. Add the remaining ingredients and mix well.

4. Fill the loaf tin and bake for 55–60 minutes.

5. Set aside to cool before turning out onto a wire rack to cool completely.

BITTERSWEET ORANGE, CHOCOLATE, AND POMEGRANATE

Serves 4

The combination of pomegranate and orange with rosewater and dark chocolate is delicious. This dish can be made before your guests arrive and it's extremely good for you.

3 oranges

1 pomegranate

½ bunch mint, chopped

¼ cup rosewater

1 teaspoon pomegranate molasses

1¼ ounces dark chocolate

METHOD

1. Remove the peel and pith from the oranges and divide into segments.

2. Remove the seeds from the pomegranate and mix the two fruits together in a bowl.

3. Add the mint.

4. Combine the rosewater with the pomegranate molasses and pour over the fruit and mint. Serve in individual dishes with a few dark chocolate shavings over the top of each.

BAKED PERSIMMON STUFFED WITH CASHEWS AND APRICOTS

The mild flavor of persimmons in contrast with the sharp apricot is perfect in these baked persimmons. We suggest you serve this dessert after quite a light main meal and use small fruits as the dish is quite filling.

¼ cup raw cashews, roasted and chopped

6 dried apricot halves, cut into small pieces

2 tablespoons cashew nut spread

4 firm Fuyu persimmons

low-fat yogurt, to serve

METHOD

1. Preheat the oven to 350°F.

2. Combine the roasted cashews, apricots, and nut spread into a paste.

3. Cut the stalks off the persimmons and use an apple corer to remove the center from each persimmon.

4. Stuff the cashew and apricot paste into the center of the persimmons.

5. Cover each individually with foil and place in a baking tray filled with 1 inch of water. Bake in the oven for 25–30 minutes.

6. Serve with low-fat natural yogurt.

Note: *Select persimmons with green caps that are free from bruises and firm to the touch. Ripe persimmons range in color from pale orange to deep red-orange, depending upon the time of season and the variety. They will keep out of the refrigerator for up to 5 days.*

OTHER ULYSSES PRESS BOOKS

Beyond the Master Cleanse: The Year-Round Plan for Maximizing the Benefits of The Lemonade Diet
Tom Woloshyn, $12.95

Millions of people have experienced the many health benefits that result from the Master Cleanse detox. *Beyond the Master Cleanse* shows how to maintain and extend those health gains for months or even years.

The Complete Master Cleanse: A Step-by-Step Guide to Maximizing the Benefits of The Lemonade Diet
Tom Woloshyn, $13.95

Fasting while drinking a lemonade-like blend of clear spring water, cayenne pepper and citrus juice has proven to be a safe, simple and yet powerful way to cleanse the body of toxins. This book goes beyond basic information on how to do the cleanse — which can be learned in minutes — by guiding readers step by step through the entire cleansing process.

The GI Mediterranean Diet: The Glycemic Index-Based Life-Saving Diet of the Greeks
Dr. Fedon Alexander Lindberg, $14.95

Mediterranean cuisine and GI dieting are a proven match made in culinary heaven. This book shows readers how the Old World's most celebrated foods can keep you lean, young and living a longer and healthier life.

The Easy GL Diet Handbook: Lose Weight with the Revolutionary Glycemic Load Program
Dr. Fedon Alexander Lindberg, $10.00

Using these more accurate and sensible GL scores, *The Easy GL Diet Handbook* offers a plan for healthy weight loss and reduced risk of diabetes that's easier to follow. It also includes numerous foods that the Atkins, South Beach, and GI diets wrongly consider "off-limits."

The GL Cookbook and Diet Plan: A Glycemic Load Weight-Loss Program with Over 150 Delicious Recipes
Nigel Denby, $12.95

Offers a vast selection of GL-scored recipes so dieters can choose dishes they love while following a proven program for permanent weight loss without hunger.

The Juice Fasting Bible: Discover the Power of an All-Juice Diet to Restore Good Health, Lose Weight and Increase Vitality
Dr. Sandra Cabot, $12.95

Offering a series of quick and easy juice fasts, this book provides a reader-friendly approach to an increasingly popular, alternative health practice.

The Simple 0-to-10 GI Diet: Lose Weight with the Easy Food-Scoring System Based on the Glycemic Index
Azmina Govindji & Nina Puddefoot, $12.95

By simplifying the scoring system and creating an easy-to-follow plan, this handbook offers a no-hassle program to lose weight and maintain a healthy long-term diet.

To order these books call 800-377-2542 or 510-601-8301, fax 510-601-8307, e-mail ulysses@ulyssespress.com, or write to Ulysses Press, P.O. Box 3440, Berkeley, CA 94703. All retail orders are shipped free of charge. California residents must include sales tax. Allow two to three weeks for delivery.

ABOUT THE AUTHORS

Joanna McMillan Price is a certified nutritionist and dietitian with a PhD in nutritional science from the University of Sydney. She is a popular media spokesperson with regular appearances on TV and radio, and is the nutrition expert for Australia's *Today* show. Joanna has authored/coauthored several previous books including *Reality Food*, *The Low GI Diet*, and *The Low GI Diet Cookbook*; she is a health writer for the magazine *Life etc*; and she writes a regular column, "Ask the Food Doctor," for *Slimming & Health* magazine. A popular nutrition presenter, Joanna regularly lectures to general practitioners, nurse practitioners, fitness instructors, and the general public. Originally from Scotland, Joanna emigrated to Australia in 1999 and now lives in Sydney with husband Michael, sons Oliver and Lewis, and Standard Schnauzer Tosca. You can find Joanna online at www.joannamcmillanprice.com.

Judy Davie is a nutrition and food writer and the author of *The Food Coach* (Penguin) and *Read the Label* (Random House). After studies in psychology, food as medicine, and macrobiotic cooking, she identified a gap in the market beyond what was offered by nutritionists and dietitians and started her own business, The Food Coach, a personal-training service in healthy eating. Combining her talents in the kitchen with nutritious food, Judy has written a popular weekly recipe section in *The Sunday Telegraph* and currently also writes a column for *Everyday Food* and *Healthy Life*. Visit Judy on her popular website www.thefoodcoach.com.au, a source of over 800 healthy recipes and numerous articles and tips on healthy eating and well-being.